Welcome to the Wealthy Fit Pro Series

The fitness industry is beautifully flawed. It simultan~
transforms lives and chews up and spits ou~   ~e
agents. If you want to stick arou~~
certification programs don't te~
necessary for success.

The *Wealthy Fit Pro* books gather t~   ~t minds in the global
fitness industry to bring you the guidance you need at the lowest
price possible. You hold in your hands the first title in this series:
Starting Your Career. My goal is not to tell you what to do in every
situation. Instead, this book will show you how to navigate each
stage of your career, from certification to landing a job to continuing
education. We'll talk about getting clients, building programs, and
developing multiple income streams to pad your bottom line.

I took this project on because when starting my career I felt alone.
I was lucky to come across mentors and read the right books at the
right time. If we want to make the world a better, healthier place,
it starts with passionate fit pros like you. You have the potential to
change lives, but it won't happen if you can't make the money that
you deserve.

I'm happy you're here and excited for your career. Welcome, and let's
dig in!

—Coach Jon

*P.S. This book is the beginning. I'd love to connect with you more. Feel free
to friend me on my personal Facebook page at **theptdc.com/fb** and send
me a message anytime. My entire team and I are here for you.*

Also by Jonathan Goodman and the Personal Trainer Development Center

Books

Ignite the Fire: The Secrets to Building a Successful Personal Training Career (Revised, Updated, and Expanded)

Personal Trainer Pocket Book: A Handy Reference for All Your Daily Questions

Viralnomics: How to Get People to Want to Talk About You

The Highly Wealthy Online Trainer box set:
Book 1: *Habits of Highly Wealthy Online Trainers*
Book 2: *Marketing Breakthroughs of Highly Wealthy Online Trainers*

All titles and an updated book list available at
theptdc.com/store.

Courses & Certifications

Online Trainer Academy
A comprehensive certification in online training.
theptdc.com/ota

Advanced Marketing Resource

Fitness Marketing Monthly — The Complete Collection
theptdc.com/fmm

FREE GIFT

Read (and Hear) Your Wealthy Fit Pro Guide Anywhere!

We want all fit pros to have easy and constant access to the best career guidance. That's why we created a special deal: To accompany the WFPG print edition you hold in your hand, we'll give you the eBook and audiobook absolutely free.

To get your free eBook and audiobook for *The Wealthy Fit Pro's Guide to Starting Your Career*, go to: theptdc.com/wfpg-syc

Enjoy with my compliments

–Coach Jon

Copyright ©2019 by J. Goodman Consulting Inc.

All rights reserved. No part of this publication may be reproduced, distributed, or transmitted in any form or by any means, without the prior written permission of J. Goodman Consulting Inc.

The Wealthy Fit Pro's Guide to Starting Your Career
ISBN: 9781070225357

Cover and interior book design by Growler Media

Bulk order discounts are available for fitness centers, education companies, academic institutions, and mentorships. Please inquire by emailing support@theptdc.com with subject line "bulk book order."

The Wealthy Fit Pro's Guide to

STARTING YOUR CAREER

JONATHAN GOODMAN

CONTENTS

———

INTRODUCTION

Welcome to the fitness industry. We're excited to have you. Now that you're here, it's time to learn the steps you need to take to set yourself up for a fitness career in line with your hopes, goals, and aspirations.

Since 2011, I've been helping personal trainers change the way they run their businesses. If you're looking for a different kind of fitness career — one that will help you work more effectively and efficiently and that is personally, professionally, and financially satisfying — then you're in the right place.

So, why this book? Well, after selling tens of thousands of copies of my first book, Ignite the Fire: The Secrets to Building a Successful Personal Training Career, I did a number of group chats and Q & A sessions with new trainers who had bought the book. They had many questions, and what I found was that the questions were quite often, frankly, bad questions.

The new trainers focused on the wrong things.

They asked questions like,

> *"What should I read?"*

instead of the more important question,

> *"How should I read?"*

because it's not just the quality of material but also the consumption and application that count.

Plus, these well-intentioned and passionate coaches wanted to know,

> *"How can I get as many people to buy my training as possible?"*

instead of asking,

> *"How can I build systems in my business to encourage clients to approach me, asking to train?"*

We live in an information-rich world where anything you want to know is at your fingertips, but one skill is vital: **You must be able to ask good questions**. A bad question will yield an answer that leads you astray.

I realized that new personal trainers needed full and unbiased answers to their biggest questions from somebody acting independently, not associated with a large certifying body. The truth is certs have lots of problems. I can't sugarcoat it. Certification is big business, and too often it operates as a factory line, pumping out not-yet-qualified trainers ill-prepared for a fitness career. Certification rarely equals qualification.

This problem isn't unique to the fitness industry. Few new graduates are ready for the workforce. Even an accountant who just passed her regulatory exam isn't ready to jump into the job, full-fledged. This accountant may have the technical knowledge, but she can't possibly have the requisite experience to know what to do in every situation.

That's why I feel something is needed to bridge the gap, helping newly certified trainers become qualified.

Graduating from frying pan to fire

It all began in 2007 — my first-ever client was a 16-year-old male who wanted to gain muscle. Cool, I could help with that. That was my background.

My second client, a 67-year-old female, had a torn ACL and arthritis so bad that she could barely grip a dumbbell. I was 21 years old, had an honors degree in kinesiology, and had been a certified trainer since I was 18, having spent three years managing the university gym throughout my studies. The only people I really knew how to train were myself and other university students.

Unlike accounting and many other industries, new trainers are thrown into the fire from day one. Sink or swim (or burn, as it were). And because they lack mentors, who should be a part of any gym's onboarding program, many fitness pros sink.

At this point, you may know how to train one type of client — the kind who desires a transformation similar to the one you went through. You won't know how to train every type of client. But you'll be expected to do just that.

My rude awakening happened when I walked into the assessment room as a bright-eyed 21-year-old trainer to greet the 67-year-old grandmother of three. I remember being nervous, sweating despite the gym's overpowering air conditioning, fully aware that I was not qualified. But there I was, and there she was, and I said hello, and we were off. Sink or swim, right? Nothing to do now but smile and take this woman's health into my hands.

While I did work with more-experienced trainers, I didn't have the type of support I needed. I also didn't know where to look for that support, which was really the biggest issue. I was lucky in that my club had management that was (and still is) committed to educating and supporting its new trainers, but that's rare. Most of the time you're expected to cut your own path.

It starts, but doesn't end, with your certification

Certifications alone don't prepare trainers. Even those that do include adequate practical experience skimp on the business side. Most countries don't even regulate trainer certification. Anybody can produce a cert and declare a trainer "certified."

This has two effects. The first is that many certifications opt for easy-and-cheap over valuable. The second is that the good certs, the ones that do adequately prepare trainers, are forced to compete with questionable companies who undercut their prices and "certify" trainers in less time. New trainers are likely to opt for these less expensive shortcuts over more involved certs. Cheaper? Easier? That's just human nature.

Some certs take one, two, or even three years to complete. Others take a weekend. Heck, some companies are so irresponsible that you can register a dog to get certified (I've done it*).

Certification companies make most of their money via continuing education or accessory certs that they try to sell to their students on an ongoing basis. There's nothing wrong with this, but the way companies present the continuing education makes it appear as if it's the only choice for the unsuspecting fitness pro to continue his or her career. That simply isn't true.

Everything comes with bias, including this book

To grow, you must consume information, and to do that properly, you must assess the quality and the source. Everything comes with bias that should be taken into consideration. Most free information is produced by somebody who will try to sell you something. That includes this book.

I want to tell you about my background and my bias.

The dog got a passing grade of 79 percent on the test. You should've seen him barking with excitement when his certificate arrived in the mail. We gave him so many treats that day.

Please consider this before taking action on any of the advice that follows.

My company works independently. I have no affiliation with any certification company. However, in 2016 I formed the first-ever certification for online trainers through an offshoot of my company called the Online Trainer Academy. Since 2011, I have been publishing free information on my website, the Personal Trainer Development Center (theptdc.com), and have published multiple books for trainers at all stages of their careers.

My goal with this book is twofold: The first is to help you at the beginning of your career by giving you the guidance I wish I had back then. That's the altruistic goal. The second is more strategic and selfish. My hope is that this book will help you so much that, as you progress throughout your career, you will keep coming back to learn from me and my team by investing in whatever book, resource, newsletter, or event is most applicable to you at the time.

With that said, I will never produce fitness equipment, sell supplements, or recommend one type of training over another. The scientific method works by assuming that a hypothesis is true until proven wrong. Said differently: Something can be true 1,000 times, but the first time it's proven to be untrue, any person with integrity must pivot and change course.

By building a business that relies on the sale of

a specific brand of fitness equipment, dietary supplement, or type of training style, the creator is forced to cherry-pick sources and shelter his or her audience. Even if proven wrong, the business is forced to ignore any disproving theories to the detriment of any observer and society's progress in general.

Pulitzer Prize-winning author Upton Sinclair, in his book *I, Candidate for Governor: And How I Got Licked*, wrote,

"It is difficult to get a man to understand something when his salary depends on his not understanding it."

Say, for example, a company is selling a functional training cert. Obviously the information it includes on its website and the other information it shares are going to claim that functional exercise, and mobility, and post-rehab, and things like that, are the end-all. This is not necessarily a bad thing. This is what the company does. This is what it sells and what it believes in. That's its bias. You must take this into account.

This is getting fun. Let's keep going.

You're an entrepreneur now

Even if you work for a club, you're responsible for your own business. If you are given clients, then it's up to you to keep them. No gym in the world will continue feeding you clients unless you can retain and renew them. At some point you'll be expected to generate new business.

This is why you need to develop the mindset of an entrepreneur. Training clients is important, but so is generating business, taking care of your finances, establishing multiple income streams, and, over time, creating a reputation for exceptional service.

To start, we're going to get back to basics and talk about how to learn. From there we'll talk programming and how to master it. After that, you'll learn all about discovering your niche, selling training, marketing yourself, continuing your education, and, finally, making more money by developing multiple income streams.

It comes down to this: You're on your own. You must forge your own path. Fitness is one of the most profitable and fulfilling industries. But if you're not careful, it can chew you up and spit you out faster than you can say myofibrillar hypertrophy.

I'm here to be your sherpa, guiding you as you strive to reach this beautifully flawed industry's highest peaks. I can't give you all of the information you'll need. That's impossible. Instead, I'll arm you with the type of thinking that you need, and tell you where to find the best tools and resources as you progress on this journey.

Let's dive in.

CHAPTER 1

Read Up
The "How" Is More Important Than the "What"

You're starting out, you're ready to launch, you want everything to just move. I know that feeling. But one of the most important things I learned — and wish I'd known it when I was starting out — is the need to keep learning every single day. Sure, you've been educated, you have certifications. Now you just need experience, right? Sorry. Continual development is paramount to enhancing your career — on day one, day two, and every day after that.

What counts as "development?" While additional certifications and training are good, reading is what will set you apart. But not all reading is equal and, as you'll soon find out, how much time you set aside to read, what you read, and, more important, how you read makes all the difference.

First, let me tackle the easy part: how much. I generally advise trainers to read a minimum of one hour a day, Monday to Friday, and to make up for lost time on the weekend. This is, of course, not set in stone, but it's a good guideline. While it may seem like a lot, making time for reading and not playing useless games on your phone will have you leapfrogging your competition.

The rule of reading a minimum of one hour, Monday to Friday, and making up for lost time on the weekend, gives you a small goal to hit. It's reasonable, it's attainable, and it's something that most people can do. If that seems like way too much, try 30 minutes a day, Monday to Friday, and make up for lost time on the weekend — whatever is reasonable for you, based on your life. (And yes, you can listen to audiobooks as well.) It doesn't even have to be 30 minutes at once. A few minutes while waiting for a bus and a few more when your client is late for his session all add up.

To make yourself accountable, write "Monday" through "Friday" on a sheet of paper and track your reading time every day. If you weren't able to get it done on a particular day, make a note for that day to catch up on the weekend. Just be sure not to miss a day — when you do, it's easy for a couple of weeks to pass with no reading/study time.

Choosing what to read

So you know you're going to read. Now, what should you read? There are two categories:

1. Business
2. Fitness

Spend about 50 percent of your time on each. Understand that this time is for professional development, not personal interests. It's easy to fall into the trap of believing that you're studying for your clients when you're simply reading fitness and nutrition info that's interesting to you. Only you can determine whether this is the case, but I will say that most clients fall in the beginner-to-intermediate category and would benefit much more from you becoming a better coach than you learning about some obscure new exercise or in-vogue workout protocol.

Trust me: As you continue in your career, you'll discover that business development is just as important as fitness or nutrition. In addition to growing your business, an understanding of marketing psychology will also make you a better coach. Aside from building your business, which is super important, your ability to get your client to want to do the workout is just as, if not more, important than the workout itself. And that takes marketing.

Get the most from your reading

Here are two strategies to better absorb what you read:

1. Create a Study Group

Forming a study group of four to six trainers (ideally

those who are relatively new to the job) can make all the difference. Aside from the networking benefit, this small group can agree on a book to read and come up with questions, talking points, drills to practice, and more.

I don't remember how it came about, but back in the day I was part of an optional weekly study group. Every Friday afternoon around 1:30 p.m. at Body + Soul Fitness, the gym where I worked in Toronto, we had an open invite for trainers from the neighborhood to meet and learn and grow with one another. It was casual — anybody could show up and bring friends.

We talked, tried different exercises, practiced facilitated stretching on each other, and, if anybody had learned something that past week, he or she was free to teach the group.

THE BEST WAY TO LEARN IS TO TEACH

Teaching forces you to break down a concept and communicate it simply enough so that it can be understood by others. When you teach, you end up with a greater understanding of the concept. Always look for opportunities to teach.

This study group can morph into a "mastermind group," something I'll talk about later in this book. For now, know that a mastermind group is a group of like-minded trainers who you meet with to brainstorm and share ideas.

2. *Study in the Gym*

The second method of studying is to do it on the gym floor. Very early in my career, I was reading *Facilitated Stretching* by Bob McAtee, a book about partner-assisted stretching. I wanted to practice what I was I reading, so I took the book into the gym the next day.

Walking around the gym, highlighted book in hand, I found it easy to approach and ask people on the floor if they were interested in a free stretch at the end of their workouts. I showed them the book and said I wanted to practice some of the techniques I was learning.

Not only did I get hands-on practice about what I was reading, but it was also an easy way to meet members, showcase my skills, and set myself apart from other trainers. In addition, busy begets busy. If you're working with people on the floor, curious onlookers don't know that you're giving a free session. The more that you're on the floor working with people, the more other people will notice you and see you engaged and in demand. And they in turn will want to work with you.

One of the people I stretched that day became a client. I'm not saying you'll be able to convert clients right away. But after I stretched him, we'd chat every time he came into the gym. Soon after, when he was ready for a trainer, he hired me.

Understand the rules of logic

Reading turns you into a trustworthy and knowledgeable source of information. You must combine this knowledge with an understanding of the rules of logic. A lot of people in this industry will claim things as facts that may or may not be so. All professionals have two responsibilities:

1. Don't be an "InstaTrainer." Just because you saw a nice exercise on social media doesn't mean the exercise is something you need to try with a client. It may be. But you shouldn't solely rely on materials your clients have access to for your education and knowledge.

That said, sometimes it can be helpful to study materials prepared for the mass market and geared toward your particular training audience. In a later chapter of this book, you'll learn about the importance of using the right words and phrases to get the requisite initial buy-in from clients, meeting them where they are so that you can take them where they want to go. These materials just shouldn't comprise all of your study time.

2. Seek out a wide variety of resources — especially those that you initially disagree with, and read and study those while respecting that they have bias. You can learn more from somebody who is successful —

and whom you disagree with — than from any other source, but it requires open-mindedness. It's easy to get engaged in groups, both online and offline, that simply reinforce what you already know or believe. If you aren't willing to challenge your belief system, you won't grow.

The "Filter Bubble" and how it affects what you see online

Let's take a moment to get a better handle on what I just said about challenging your belief systems. It's crucial to understand how social media feeds, online searches, and online communities form and operate as part of something called the "filter bubble," so I'm going to go off on a tangent here and give you some background about it. Only when you understand how the algorithms have been built to feed you information you already agree with can you build in the systems to see past it.

Consider: When you use a free platform like Facebook or Google, you are not the consumer. You are the product being sold. Information that you input into the system by way of things you view, click on, and post and people you interact with are all being tracked, packaged, and sold to advertisers. This compiled information gets sent to data companies, organized, mixed with other data from things like frequent buyer programs, and sold to the highest bidder.

What I just described is a basic overview of how companies like Facebook and Google develop their ad networks. You can't do anything about this except stop using these platforms. It is what it is.

In addition to advertisements, this data is also used to provide you with better search or, as I like to call it, reverse search. You and I could type the exact same thing into Google and get different results. What you see in your Facebook feed is different from what I see in mine. The algorithms that manage these systems are getting more powerful by the day and know what you want to see before you even know to search it.[*]

Reverse search exists for two reasons:

The better a platform is at providing you what you want to hear and who you want to hear from, the better the chance that you will keep coming back.

You will buy more.

For a free platform to operate, it needs to be monetized. To make money, it shows you ads paid for by companies wanting you to buy things. If you don't buy things, the ads are worthless and companies pay less for them. As a result, the free platform optimizes everything about it in the hopes that you will click on the advertisements contained within to buy stuff so that advertisers pay more.

Ever log in to Facebook and see something you're interested in or were thinking about and thought it was creepy that Facebook knew to show it to you? This is why.

TO READ NEXT:

If this section is interesting to you and you want to know how to use this knowledge to increase your impact on social media, buy a copy of *Viralnomics: How to Get People to Want to Talk About You.*

You won't learn "the best time to post on Facebook," because that doesn't really matter. Instead, you'll learn the timely, yet timeless principles to help you win at social not just today, but far into the future even as the social landscape changes. **Buy the paperback directly from our store at theptdc.com/store** or the Kindle or audio version from Amazon.

We don't buy things from people we don't like, and we don't buy things when the messages we see contradict our pre-existing belief patterns. One way these free platforms maximize conversions is to produce a filter bubble that's unique to each user based on actions they took in the past. Each user sees things and people they like, and, as a result, they buy more.

Phew, that got intense for a second. But why does it all matter?

It matters because the system is designed to show you things you already agree with. The effect is that your belief system isn't challenged and, even if you do see something that you don't agree with, it's surrounded by so many things that are connected to your existing beliefs that you probably won't engage.

Fight this in order to stay open to other ideas — even those that may contradict what you believe. Here's my challenge: If you haven't changed your mind about something, or haven't been exposed to something that opposes your current line of thought in the last two weeks, I want you to pick up a magazine that you've never read before or click onto a website that you've never visited or reach out to a coach you've never met and ask him or her a question.

It's important to gather as much information as possible to come to your own conclusions while being open enough to change your mind if proven wrong. You want to prevent something called *confirmation bias*: the tendency to see things in a way that supports our pre-existing belief patterns.

All of this being said, I'm also a realist.

There are limitations to science when we're talking about fitness, and it's why you should accept very little as absolute "fact." We simply cannot do the type of testing on humans to conclusively establish, for example, which type of workout is the absolute best. People are too different. There are too many variables to try to control. My job is not to tell you what to think, but how to approach thinking.

Become a first-rate analyzer

Knowing how to analyze content means never reading something and simply nodding your head. Dig into it. When deciding whether to pay attention to an information source, always ask whether the person, company, or brand is built around a particular ideal, hook, or belief that limits it from changing directions (or admitting that the belief is wrong). If a business is based around a particular ideology, the purveyors of the information are forced to cherry-pick research, insulate followers from information that doesn't jibe with what they say, and continue to publish one-sided views.

Think of people who build their brand off ideas like ketogenic diets, paleo, a particular supplement, or a specific piece of fitness equipment. None of these concepts may be bad, but you can't blindly trust information coming from them or their supporters. Somebody who sells nutrition advice based on the paleo diet has reason to promote supportive evidence and discredit or ignore unsupportive evidence.

Curate your TBR list

Every successful person I know has a long "TBR" — as in, "to be read" — list of books, articles, links, and more. Back in the pre-digital day of paper-only, that meant endlessly stashed books, magazines, journals, and photocopies, and folks would say, "My TBR pile is taller than I am." That's your goal in today's digital-and-maybe-some-paper realm. Curate a healthy TBR pile and you'll always have some content to tap into.

Meanwhile, you now know to question what you read and consume, depending on who it's coming from, and why it's being disseminated. As I said earlier in this chapter, you should focus on material that will help you with your clients, and/or build your business. According to Mark Young, the owner of Christ Centered Fitness, a remote training company operating out of Hamilton, Canada, you should consider three things when determining what to read.

1. Is this content relevant to your business or day-to-day activities with clients?

The newest exercise variation may be exciting and interesting, but is it relevant to your programming? Maybe. Maybe not. I mean, new exercises look really cool and get us seen-it-all trainers excited.

But most of your clients are beginners. They need to learn basic movement patterns. So, is doing a single-leg squat with a twist on the end of it really going to be all that important for them?

Probably not.

2. Is the content valid?

I've just shown you how to analyze the legitimacy of the information source, but I want to add one more factor to consider: Is the entity putting out the content using "logical fallacies" to make their information appear more valid?

Example: You see people debate things all the time. I don't necessarily mean a formal debate, where people argue directly with each other. Facebook posts that stir up comments are arguably (see what I did there?) the most common form of debate today. When you know how to recognize logical fallacies, it's easier to qualify the information being presented.

There are a few logical fallacies to look for:

The Straw Man Attack
This is when one side argues a point, based on only part of the issue at hand, or a different issue altogether. An example was when I let two trainers write articles on the subject of whether poor sitting posture contributes to pain. One argued that it does; the other, that it did not.

One writer used studies of participants' standing posture to argue her point, but the debate was about whether sitting posture affects pain. That's a straw man attack — basing your conclusions on things that are irrelevant to the point being debated. [⚭]

The Ad Hominem Attack
This is where one side resorts to personal attacks or attempts to take down a person's character, as opposed

⚭ *For a full breakdown on how to analyze fitness research, go to* ***theptdc.com/research***.

to arguing the facts. Name-calling falls under this category.

In both the case of the straw man and ad hominem attacks, the use of a logical fallacy doesn't mean the person using it isn't worth listening to. However, when you see a straw man or ad hominem attack, you should be aware of it — and question the person's intent and the validity of the information he or she is offering.

3. Does the content fit into your model or system?

The exercises you have your clients perform must be the best option for them — not the newest or most exciting. So, is that single-leg squat variation you just learned better than whatever existing movement you would have used in that particular situation for your client? If it is, and you're sure, plug it in and eliminate the old. If not, figure out where and how this new fancy single-leg variation may fit in somewhere else — or throw it out the window.

When you get a new piece of information — like a new exercise, new way of eating, or a new way of marketing yourself — I suggest you ask the following four questions:

1. How does this information fit my system?
2. How is it better?
3. What kind of client will benefit from it?
4. Where could it go in an individual program?

Your reading and studying time, with these fallacies

and questions in mind, must be non-negotiable. There is nothing that you can do to further your career that is more important than this. Stick to it. If you do, you'll progress faster than the rest of your cohorts. If not, you'll stagnate.

"But Coach Jon, I still want to know *what* to read."

No problem. One way is to pay attention to online chatter when coaches you admire talk about what they're reading. Also, and more immediate, I maintain a reading list of the top business and fitness books on the Personal Trainer Development Center website.

For an up-to-date list of book recommendations, go to **theptdc.com/book-list**.

THE TAKEAWAY

Spend at least an hour a day, Monday through Friday, reading books that will help make you a better trainer. Analyze what you read so that you can determine its validity and how to apply it to your clients and your business.

CHAPTER 2

Find a Job
How to I.D. the Perfect Workplace for You

Where to work used to be a simple question for fit pros. After completing your certification, the only option was to find a job at the local gym. Things have changed.

Nowadays, countless options are available to you from big box gyms to more boutique studios to remote work and everything in between. What you'll learn in this t is that there isn't one capital-B Best place to work, but there is probably a right fit for you right now. Over time your needs may change. Let this chapter help you decide the perfect fit not just for your financial goals, but also for your personal success and fulfillment.

First things first — do you know who you want to work with?

New trainers typically are in one of two positions:

- You already know what type of clientele you want to work with.

- You have no idea.

There are a few reasons why you may be sure of the type of clientele that you want to work with. Let's say that, for example, training is your second, third, or even fourth career, and you wish to train the 40-to-50-plus-year-old crowd. That's a good market, and you'd be well-suited for it. There are countless other examples. Maybe you were a competitive hockey player and want to train young hockey players.

If this is the case, where to work becomes an easier decision. But there are still some factors to consider before you launch your job search.

The obvious point: If you do know what kind of clientele you want to work with, look for a facility that focuses on them. If you want to train young hockey players, go to a facility that trains hockey players or young athletes.

And if you want to train older adults, say 40-, 50-, or 60-year-olds, or even older, you'd probably look for a boutique studio that focuses on that crowd, instead of a big box gym where most members are in their 20s or 30s.

I should add that although you may think you're sure who you want to train, your preference could change, and pursuing a job at a facility centered around one type of client could pigeonhole you into a career path that is less than ideal.

It's hard to know who you love training unless you train a lot of different types of clients. Enjoying a certain lifestyle or sport can be very different from training others for that lifestyle or sport.

So you want to train pro athletes and celebrities...

A lot of young trainers aspire to train public figures: Pro or elite-level athletes, actors, musicians, and more. Let's talk about that. I'll give you a few examples from my own training life because I wanted to train athletes when I began my career. With a degree in kinesiology and the Certified Strength and Conditioning Specialist (CSCS) designation from the National Strength and Conditioning Institute (NSCA), I was well-suited to this and quickly became a go-to in my neighborhood for young athletes.

One of my past clients is now a second-line center in the National Hockey League as of this writing and just signed a $9 million contract. I helped him with his conditioning for the NHL combine when he was a teenager. It's been fun to watch his career progress. I also trained Canada's top jazz singer for many years. Helping her get out of pain and watching her get a standing ovation after her performance at Massey Hall, the Holy Grail of music venues in Canada, was a joy. Throughout my career I also had the pleasure of working with multiple Olympians and actors.

All of these clients were dedicated, hard-working, and fulfilling to train. They also taught me that I didn't want to train more than one or two celebrities or athletes at a time. It's sexy to train celebrities and athletes, but, as anybody who trains a lot them will attest, it's often more trouble than it's worth once the day-to-day settles in.

These "star" clients have demanding schedules that change fast. The seasonality of sport, filming schedules, and music tours cut into training. From a financial standpoint, you're not making more from training these clients than you are from the average Joe and Jane. The difference is that they aren't around as much and create holes in your schedule. Working with off-season hockey players is great until the season starts and you're left with an empty schedule. Working with a musician is awesome until that musician goes on tour in Asia for three months and you don't have a client 9:30 to 10:30 am Monday, Wednesday, or Friday for three months, and at the end of the tour, you need to have that spot free for her so that she can recommence her training.*

If you're in the second position, where you are not sure yet what type of client you want to work with (or if I just changed your mind and you now realize that maybe you aren't quite sure anymore), then your best bet is to work with as many different people from as many different walks of life as possible. That's experience you can use.

---

* *Hypothetically speaking, of course.*

Prioritize learning opportunities above all else (for now)

No matter what kind of clientele you hope to train, I recommend looking for a facility that offers a continuing education program and has open-minded staff and management. Even if this is your second career, it's important that you start off on the right foot and choose a place that gives you an opportunity to grow. You want a place that understands that new trainers need mentoring and support and that the job isn't a competition. There are plenty of clients to go around. The minute you witness staff or management operating with a scarcity mindset, run. A good facility will have somebody available to support you and answer questions.

This may mean that you don't pick the gym that pays the most. Becoming "qualified" means prioritizing learning — at least for now. You may take a hit in income at first, but your earning potential will grow with experience. More knowledge now means more money later.

Another thing to watch out for: Gyms that have the marketing clout to feed you clients usually pay the worst. Facilities that pay a lot will expect you to drive your own business which, at this point, you may or may not be able to do.

Regardless, it's early in your career and your focus should be on working with a lot of people. Opt for less pay (if you can afford it) if it means that the gym will put you in front of more people. You can always move to a facility that pays more later, once you have more experience.

What makes a gym the right place for you?

Remember, gyms are businesses. They're trying to attract new clients and good trainers. They'll try to make themselves as attractive as possible to you. Don't let a shiny new thing derail your overall strategy. Regardless of whether you know what types of clients you want to work with, it's important to keep your options open. A gym based around a "hook" or fad or one specific type of training may seem cutting edge, but this isn't a good idea early on. You simply don't know what you like yet. Fads flame out, shiny things grow dull, and the same old boring stuff is usually what works best anyway.

So what's the "perfect" fit for you? (Hint: There are no perfect fits). Let's look at some of the most popular options and the pros and cons of each. Then I'll give you some questions to help you determine whether a particular facility is right for you.

Big box gyms

Big box gyms, or commercial gyms, get a lot of hate. Stories of mistreating trainers, broken promises, and abysmally low pay are all too common. Still,

I recommend most trainers start their careers at one of them. Just make sure that the club has good management and good mentors available.

You should interview a gym just as much as they are interviewing you. Ask them about continuing education funds and availability of mentors. Even more important: If you're considering working there, I always recommend joining the gym for a week or two first. Spend time working out there. Watch the trainers for their energy, how they create atmosphere, and if they seem to have good morale and smile a lot. Can you see yourself spending a lot of long days there?

Many big box gyms have sales goals that trainers need to meet, both to keep their jobs and to advance in pay. Be sure to inquire about sales goals and make sure you understand and are comfortable with them before signing your contract.

Big box gyms have a lot of marketing pull and usually a large client base for you to work with off the bat. You'll have access to different equipment and clientele with different goals and limitations. I repeat this point multiple times because I cannot overstate its importance.

Boutique facilities

My first job and my entire full-time training career happened at the boutique training studio Body + Soul Fitness in Toronto. It focuses on high-end personal training. When I started, the company had a single location, but it has since expanded to multiple locations throughout Toronto.

"Boutique" generally means smaller training facilities that have one to three locations, are local to an area, are privately owned, and focus on one type of clientele (like hockey players, for example, or maybe affluent clients who want a private training experience).

The club paid more than the big box facilities around town, and it had a fantastic continuing education program (it still does). But it was a difficult place for new trainers because it didn't have a large existing client base or marketing budget for new trainers to pull from. Newbies had to develop their own clientele. This wasn't easy, especially if they were trying to develop themselves at the same time.

This kind of environment was great for me, but it may not be good for a lot of new trainers. The pros? You usually get higher pay and more attention from management than you would at big box gyms. The major cons: You're in charge, at least to a certain extent, of developing your own business. And you won't be exposed to much of a variety of clientele.

Also important to consider, but not necessarily a pro or a con, is that boutique studios are quieter and more private. For years, I spent 12- to 14-hour days in a gym that had a total of 50 people come through in a day. I like people, just not a lot of them at once, so this suited me well. But if you're extroverted and need constant action, you'll want a facility with a lot more foot traffic.

In-home training

A lot of new trainers like the in-home option because it's easy to get your feet wet training clients in their own homes. You write a program for them, make the house call, and train them using either their own equipment or gear that you bring — and then you leave.

Financially, it seems like a great idea. There's little overhead, and you can be paid in cash. (Although you should claim everything you make and pay appropriate taxes, I've got a feeling that not all in-home trainers are 100 percent honest when reporting their income).

But here is why I don't think in-home training is a great option for most new trainers: The beginning of a career needs to be dedicated to your development. If you want to make this a sustainable, fulfilling, long-term career, you need to spend as much time as you can getting better.

In-home trainers have to build their own client list. Maybe you find your initial clientele through friends or family, or through flyers on the street — it can be done any number of ways — but often your clients will fall into similar categories. If you lose a client, the person is more difficult to replace because you've got to start from scratch, as opposed to working in a gym where you develop relationships and rapport with members over time.

Plus, more than anything, in-home training is lonely. You'll spend a lot of time driving, and in coffee shops waiting out breaks between clients or cancellations.

If you do choose to start training clients at home, I recommend that you develop a mastermind group of other in-home trainers that meets every two weeks. You can discuss your clients and any challenges you're facing with these other trainers and stave off some of the loneliness.

What are your absolutes?

Now that you know something about career options for new trainers, the next step is to write your "absolutes" and use that list to guide your decision. Some questions to ask yourself:

- What type of clientele do I want to work with? "I don't know" is a perfectly fine answer.

- What type of management do you desire? Do you need somebody to manage and guide you — even micromanage you? Do you prefer somebody who lets you do your own thing? Do you want somebody with more of an open-door policy, where you can go in and ask questions whenever you want? Or do you want somebody who will let you make your own mistakes — and who may not be as open to assisting you with every question you have?

- How much continuing education do you want to have available to you? That includes both in-house sources at the gym and funds for outside training.

- Are you willing to do your own marketing to get clients? If so, to what extent?

- How much pay do you need? Be honest with yourself here.

How much money do you really need to make?

You may be surprised that money, specifically how much money that you need to make, was not a central factor in my recommendations for choosing where to work. My belief that professional development takes priority over income in the starting stages of your career is clear, but I'm also a realist.

This is a job. You have bills. You need to eat and keep a roof over your head. That means money. How much money you need is something that I cannot answer for you. What I do know is the idea that "more is better," at this point in your career, is not necessarily true, and that type of thinking will handcuff your earning potential later on.

How much money you truly need is a problem and, like all problems, must be defined before you go looking for the best solution. Once you know how much you need, you can figure out whether a gym you're considering is in that financial ballpark — and how many hours a day it'll take to keep you there. And once you know that? You'll have a financial goal to hit and know how much time each week you'll have left over to invest in your development. In other words, you need to earn for today and work toward higher earning potential for tomorrow.

Most people won't do this. The simple equation that I'm about to share is why I was able to blast past competing trainers in my town at such a young age, finding myself at the top of the pay scale in Toronto only four years into my career. And it's why I was able to later write a book (*Ignite the Fire*) that led me to find my place in the fitness industry. It gave me the freedom to pursue that path and led to more income streams and far more personal wealth that I ever, in my wildest dreams, imagined.

It all started with defining how much money I really needed so I could make better choices with my time. Once I did this, I let go of some clients, scaled back my hours, and used that extra time to learn and build a stronger business structure to support me.

Below is what I call the "freedom number" equation, the basic calculation that I repeat in almost every one of my books and courses. It's a simple way to figure out how much money you need each month to live and, if applicable, take care of any dependents.

Revisit this equation often as your life evolves. By having a clear idea how much money you need at any one time, you easily calculate whether you are making "enough" so that you have the confidence to invest the rest of your time on personal/professional development, networking, a dream project, or anything else that will slingshot you forward.

To calculate your freedom number, start by tallying up the amount of money per month that you need to fulfill your basic needs: rent, food, funds to care for others (if applicable), and a small amount for extravagance (which I call my "do something special for my beautiful wife" fund.)

When I first created my freedom number, here's what it looked like:

> *Rent = $1,900/month
> *Food = $500/month
> *Extravagance = $200/month

My freedom number was $2,600. It was low because I didn't have any dependents and lived a low-key lifestyle. Yours may be higher, and that's fine.

Figure out what your number is. Don't worry about anybody else's.

Next, calculate your "continued funds," which means any money that you earn passively (investments, royalties, and other things that accrue with no effort from you). Don't worry if you don't have any. I didn't for a long time. I do now, and you probably will find something for yourself later, too. But I'm getting ahead of myself. We'll talk about that in the "make more money as a trainer" chapter.

Putting it all together, here's what the freedom number equation looks like:

$$\textbf{freedom number} =$$
$$\textbf{essential expenses - continued funds}$$

Once you have your freedom number, use it when interviewing to figure out whether a potential job at a gym gets you there and, if so, how many hours you need to work to hit it.

For example: If your freedom number is $3,000/month pretax and the gym pays you $20/hour, then you will need to train 150 hours/month, or 37.5 hours/week. Not impossible, but this represents a high training load and takes some time to achieve and maintain unless the gym is going to feed you a swath of clients. It also leaves very little room for error.

In an ideal world, you want to be working twenty-five to thirty client hours a week. That may not be possible with your required income and the training jobs available to you, but it's a good goal to shoot for. Anything more than thirty hours cuts into personal development time and leads to burnout.

Also keep in mind that training hours you get paid for are very different from overall working hours. Most training jobs will pay you only for the hours that you're actually with clients, so 37.5 training hours will probably mean 55- to 60-hour weeks in the gym (or more) taking into account holes in your schedule.

I can't tell you how much you need to make or whether a training job at a particular gym for a particular pay rate is good or bad. Instead, use the freedom number equation to figure out whether it will work for you and set a realistic goal for the number of clients you need each week and each month to make it happen.

The interview process

I said it before and it bears repeating: An interview goes both ways. You should interview the gym just as much as it is interviewing you. While all interviews are different, this short section will help you prep for the meeting and gather the information you need to make the right choice.

The basics:

- **Dress one step up from training gear.** Good shoes, khakis, and a collared shirt are always safe bets. Workout clothing can be fine, but it should be nice, clean, well-fitting gear with clean running shoes.

- **Confirm the meeting.** Call or email the day before to confirm, saying that you're looking forward to the interview.

- **Bring extras.** Additional copies of your resume and references are a good idea.

- **Come prepared.** Research the gym beforehand and come prepared with questions for your interviewer. A good one to ask: What, in his or her opinion, is a common skill or approach that the gym's most successful trainers share.

The day of:

- **Show up early.** Arrive 10 to 15 minutes ahead of your appointment. To make sure that you control the timing, get to that part of town earlier in the day and read in a coffee shop nearby.

- **Breath mints and deodorant.** Use 'em. Nobody wants to smell your coffee breath, especially an interviewer.

- **Everybody matters.** From the minute you walk into the gym, arm yourself with a smile, give everybody a nice hello, and try to make small talk with any reception or support staff.*

The sitdown

All gyms have different interview processes and look for different kinds of answers, so it's hard for me to give you a precise way to prepare. What I will say is that most interviewers are more interested in *how* you answer than *what* you answer.

Back in the day I would be more impressed by an interviewee confidently saying, "I don't know the

---

* When I was interviewing trainers I would ask our receptionist what she thought of each candidate. If the person didn't greet her with a nice smile and hello, it was an immediate "no." How you do one thing is how you do everything. Trainers must be engaging and approachable even when they aren't with a client. The small things, like what you do when nobody's watching, will contribute to your success as much, or more, than anything you do with a client.

answer to that," than if that person stumbled through a fake-it-til-you-make-it moment. If that same person followed up with an email later that day with the answer that he or she researched immediately after our meeting, boom, instant hire. Nobody expects you to know everything. What matters is that you're aware of what you know and willing to do the research to figure out what you don't.

To help you identify whether the gym is a good fit for you, I've included some tips and questions to ask the gym below. Pick and choose what to ask for your situation and what you want.

- What do you consider to be the current strengths (and weaknesses) of your training staff?

- What do you feel is the biggest issue facing your personal training department today?

- What are the pay and opportunities for increases, and is a wage earned only when working with clients or is there a salary as well?

- Do you provide opportunities for continuing education? What are they?

- Would it be possible to chat with one of your trainers to get his or her experience working here day-to-day?

After the interview

Handwrite a thank-you note to the person who interviewed you and put it in the mail that day.

Don't email. Write it by hand, put it in an envelope, slap a stamp on it, and put it in a mailbox. You will be the only person who does this and will immediately stand out.

The note can be basic. Copy the script below, making it specific to the person and gym if you like.

> *Dear Mr./Ms. _____,*
>
> *Thank you for your time and the opportunity to interview for a personal training position at (gym name). I really enjoyed seeing the facility and meeting you. I'm looking forward to your decision and hopefully working with you in the near future.*
>
> *—Your Name*

A quick note about insurance

Trainers need insurance. Liability insurance, for sure, and disability insurance isn't a bad idea, either. The question is: Where do you get it? It's possible that the gym where you work (or would like to work) will cover you. But be sure. Most any insurance company will have policies, and all major certification companies offer it.

You might be tempted to skimp here, and maybe you're the most careful trainer on the planet, but are you willing to risk a lawsuit for something as random as bad luck? General liability insurance will cover you if your client gets hurt by accident, like slipping and falling in the gym. What it won't cover: Negligence or overstepping your professional boundaries. But be careful. There's no official "scope of practice" for trainers, which means you could be liable with general coverage even if you do what you think is in your job description. Examples: A client has a bad reaction to your unusual nutrition plan or injures herself doing a heavy lift while fatigued. When you sign up for an insurance policy, know your coverage. Ask your insurance advisor about policies that cover liability and malpractice.

Disability insurance covers your income if you get hurt. Your livelihood depends on physical ability, so what happens if you're in a car crash and can't train for a few weeks or months? Think before you commit, however. Early in my career, I never had disability coverage because I thought the coverage was lousy (no payout until I was off for six months or more) and I had no dependents at the time. Coverage varies and you may be in a different personal situation, so decide accordingly.

THE TAKEAWAY

Carefully consider all your work options when pursuing your first job. A position that lets you train a variety of clients and offers continuing education opportunities is often the best long-term choice for a new trainer.

CHAPTER 3

Stand Out

How (and When) to Choose Your Niche

A good question: "Should I create a niche?"

Yes, you should.

A better question: "When should I create a niche?"

Let's find out.

It's important to find your niche eventually — but avoid jumping into one too soon. In the last chapter, I told you that my original career goal was to train athletes. I got my CSCS from the NSCA and worked with a few young hockey players to prep them for the National Hockey League draft. I also trained an Olympic moguls skier and an Olympic gymnast.

Even though it's what I *thought* I wanted to do, I didn't enjoy it. Later I found that I loved working with 30- to 50-year-old professionals who had back pain. Now that's the definition of "niche." It sounds weird — the polar opposite of what I thought I wanted — and yet it energized and excited me.

So how do you figure out the type of clients you'll enjoy working with?

Well, the first step is to recognize the signs smacking you in the face. When working with my athlete clients, I found myself bored. While researching, trying to get better at programming for athletes, I could hardly stay awake. I tried to read textbooks like Tudor Bompa's *Periodization for Athletic Programs* and couldn't stick with it. On the other hand, I found myself engrossed in Stuart McGill's textbook, *Low Back Disorders*.

In the section that follows, I'll give you advice on choosing a niche to maximize opportunity and profitability.

There are accessible niche markets in the tiniest of interest groups and demographics. What's most important is that you eventually focus on working with people in a way that is interesting, exciting, and energizing to you. For example, I've met a woman who only trains nudists who want outdoor workouts in the English countryside. If there's a market for English countryside nudist bootcamp workout retreats, there's a market for just about anything.

Find a subject that you want to stay up at night studying and you will always find work. Choose a niche just because you think it presents a good business opportunity and you'll grow disenchanted with it, do a poor job, and fail to drive business.

Four questions to ask when pursuing your niche

According to Elsbeth Vaino, a coach in Ottawa, Canada, and someone who has mastered her own training niche (more on that in a moment), these key questions will help you define your niche:

1. "How big is it?"
2. "What's the competition?"
3. "Do the clients you want to attract have time and money?"
4. "Do they care about what you can do for them?"

The ideal niche is:

- Big
- Underserved
- Liquid (i.e., its clients have money)

Let's take a look at a couple of niches to help illustrate how these questions work.

Say you want to create a niche serving high-end bartenders. A lot of people work in bars, so the niche is big. The niche is not particularly well-served — I don't know anybody who owns it yet. Most bartenders have midday availability because they work at night. That's perfect for most trainers. And while they aren't affluent, they generally have disposable income.

That answers the first three questions. As for whether
they care about what you can do for them? Working
at a bar is a demanding job, and bartenders must stay
fit and healthy or they can't make money. Achy knees,
backs, shoulders, and elbows are pretty common. That,
and depending on what kind of bar they work in, their
income may be largely dependent on their appearance.
These can all be selling points.

I'm having fun with this. Let's dive deeper.

A lot of male bartenders roll up their sleeves while
they work. It may be dark, but customers can see their
forearms. A training angle could be to sell them on
getting big, veiny forearms. You can also help them
develop their shoulders so their shirts fit really nice.
With any clients, your marketing should meet them
where they are to give you the opportunity to take them
where they need to go. Once you get them in the door
to work on the superficial bits, you can add in some
glute training to help reduce their achy backs because
they're on their feet so much.

Female staff may be wearing tighter shirts with either
short or no sleeves, so they may want shoulder and arm
training as well. In addition, they'll be carrying trays so
it's important to keep them strong. Like the guys, they
need glute training, and you'll want to do soft tissue
work on their calves if they wear heels a lot.

Now, understand that I'm making this up as I go. I've

jumped to many conclusions and made sweeping assumptions about gender roles. But I've been to high-end bars and seen how male and female bartenders work and dress. So while not in the least bit authoritative, this deep dive is designed to show you the kind of observational and analytical chops you should bring to the task. That's how you break down a specific client in a specific niche with the goal of strategically planning your approach.

Are you in the right niche?

Determining your niche doesn't mean that you can't change it. Track where your business is coming from, because you may be in for a surprise. Years ago Elsbeth Vaino gave a talk at an event that I hosted for my company, the Personal Trainer Development Center, where she discussed her two niches — skiing and Ultimate Frisbee.

At first glance, skiers would appear to score better in almost every way based on our four questions — a huge sport with very little competition and the clients likely have disposable time and money. And I've never met a skier who didn't want to become a better skier.

But when Elsbeth examined where her income was coming from, she got quite a surprise. Ultimate Frisbee was the big leader. She was the only game in town. Even though skiing was the bigger niche, there ended up being more competition than she originally thought, and it was hard for her to stand out.

After crunching the numbers, Elsbeth shifted her focus to being the Ultimate Frisbee expert in her community. She sponsored events, played on teams, and networked in the tight-knit community. Her business exploded. [*]

Build your expertise within a niche

Okay, you've chosen a niche. Now you want to become an expert on it. Here are your steps.

First, obtain additional education. That's obvious, isn't it? This may be a certification, or it could be a matter of seeking out experts in that field and reading their publications. If you're exploring a niche with scant information aimed at trainers, find and study materials aimed at other professionals. Personal training is still a relatively young industry, so we may lack trainer-specific materials for some niches.

Second, talk to other experts or trainers in this niche. In chapter one, I suggested creating a study group with other new trainers to help you learn. A mastermind group has a similar purpose. Why not create a mastermind group of four to six other trainers who work in the same niche? Meet every few weeks to talk about what's going on. You can share your struggles and successes.

---

*Read more about Elsbeth's experience and story in "Your Ultimate Guide to Finding the Niche to Set Yourself Apart in the Fitness Industry" at **theptdc.com/niche**.*

Your mastermind doesn't need to be local. Go online and look for people who serve the same type of niche that you do. Reach out. Get on a Skype call with them, once every month, and just talk about what's going on.

Third, interview people in your target niche. Talk to a friend who works in a bar, or take somebody from your desired niche out for coffee. Despite living in an information-abundant world, there's still no substitute for having real conversations with real people. The more the better, and this isn't something you do only when you're getting to know your niche; it should be ongoing.

Let's say you're talking to a friend who works in a bar. You may ask questions like "Do your feet hurt at night?" or "Does your back bother you?" If so, use that as you market yourself to this niche. You're not going to use trainer-speak and say, "I'm going to help strengthen your glutes, which will help stabilize your back." Instead try, "Is your back killing you because you're on your feet so much? I can help it hurt less."

No matter how passionate you are about your niche, becoming an expert on it takes time. There's no shortcut. You need to buy books, read studies, speak to a lot of people, and purchase any continuing education materials you need to make sure that you are an expert now, and into the future.

Oh, and it's not enough to say that you're an expert in something. If you're not an expert in the niche, you're offering a poor product. And great marketing with a poor product is just going to make you fail faster.

THE TAKEAWAY

Working within a niche can help you stand out from other trainers, but carefully consider which niche is right for you before you look for or create one.

CHAPTER 4

Boost Your Credentials
The Truth About Continuing Education

Now that you've got your original certification, how do you boost your credentials moving forward? There's an ever-increasing number of certifications, continuing education courses, and other opportunities to build upward from your original cert. Finding options that are right for you will save money and time, and you'll pursue the ones that will have a measurable impact on your career.

The pros and cons of certifications

First, you may not know a lot about how certifications in the fitness industry work. Personal training lacks governmental regulation just about everywhere in the world. And in places where a centralized body does exist (like the U.K. and Australia), just about anybody can apply and teach the cert as long as he or she meets some very basic criteria. This means that anybody can create a course and call it a certification. It also means that the letters behind your name, while they may make you *think* you look good, don't count for much.

In this chapter, I'll tell you about the benefits of supplemental certifications and training. After that, I'll fill you in on the best-kept secret about boosting your credentials.

Getting certified is just the beginning

A cert in no way means that you're qualified. You'll want additional training and there are a host of additional courses, sometimes called certifications, that bring genuine benefits.

A supplemental cert can be good for three things:

1. *Evidence of Advanced Knowledge*

You can become an authority on a specific subject — like "certified kettlebell instructor," or "certified old-age training specialist," or what have you. If you have a client who requires a specific kind of training, and you have a cert that covers it, the client has even more reason to justify a purchase.

A certification doesn't necessarily mean that you are any more or less prepared to help the client than somebody who did his or her own study and doesn't have the cert. However, having a cert can change the perception in your client's eyes and give a reason to choose you over somebody else. As a result, almost any supplemental certification will pay for itself quickly.

2. Potential Access to New Opportunities

Some certs are recognized in influential circles and may open doors for you. Example: The Certified Strength and Conditioning Specialist (CSCS) designation from the National Strength and Conditioning Association is a well-respected cert and more difficult to get than others.

Back in the day, I wanted to write for *Men's Health* and discovered that the editors required all fitness writers to have the CSCS designation (this has since changed). The editors needed an easy way to figure out whether someone was educated or not, and CSCS became the standard.

3. Streamlined Learning

A supplemental cert provides you with an organized way to learn about a particular subject. To me, this is the most valuable asset of a certification, but it's not unique. Many courses and education products provide this benefit, but I've found that having a certification tag associated with it generally means that the course creator is a bit more serious.

It's true that you can usually get the info you need to master a subject online. But that requires a lot of hours falling down internet rabbit holes trying to find it. If you can afford the outlay, paying somebody for neatly packaged information is a great investment because you're buying back your time.

Let's use kettlebells as an example. You could learn anything you would ever want about kettlebells by patching together free online resources: videos, articles, maybe even free courses. But a course creator has taken all of that information and saved you time by packaging it into something consumable.

Before You Buy: A deeper dive into the certification industry

As you can see, there are good reasons to acquire supplemental certs. But when you consider where to spend your valuable continuing education funds, you should understand how the certification industry *really* works.

First, certifying trainers is big business. Companies that offer baseline certifications (i.e., the cert you get when you first become a trainer) make a lot of money from follow-up certifications. So the company that initially gave you your certification will probably email the heck out of you to get you to buy more education from them.

This follow-up business is the bread and butter for these companies. In some cases, they lose money selling you your original certification (when you factor in marketing and delivery costs) hoping to make it back later. In all cases, it's in the company's best interest to insulate you from outside educational opportunities and convince you to do its courses.

I'm not saying you should avoid supplemental education sold through your original certifying company. I just don't want it to affect your continuing education decisions. If there's a course you want to do offered by somebody else, do it.

You'll find that you almost always need "CECs," or continuing education credits (sometimes called "CEUs," or continuing education units), to keep your certification current. Certification companies require you to renew your cert on a regular basis — anywhere from annually to every five years. You'll have to submit a certain number of CECs or CEUs to show that you've kept your education up-to-date.

What most trainers, even experienced ones, don't know is just how easy it is to acquire continuing education credits. Basically all types of education can be considered for CECs/CEUs. All major certifying bodies have a petition process where you can fill out a form, supply some information about your "unsanctioned" education, and get the credits that you deserve.

So don't think that you have to take courses through your original certification company or even those pre-approved by your certifying company. Typically, all you need to provide is proof of completion, with the date, a brief description, and the number of contact hours.

Buyer Beware: All courses are *not* created equal

There is rarely any official quality oversight of certs and continuing education programs. How can you tell something is on the level? Look for recommendations from people and sources you trust and try to find programs that have established a good reputation. If possible, connect with previous students before investing. Ask yourself whether the info included in that course is something you want to learn, and is it offered by somebody you want to learn from.

While most companies providing continual development to trainers are legit, I've heard lots of horror stories. The truth is, anybody can create a "course," offer coaching to trainers, and make a lot of promises. It's big business, and unfortunately, not everyone is honest. [&]

THE TAKEAWAY

Be thoughtful and selective about your continuing education and you'll truly build your qualifications — as long as you understand what supplemental certs can, and cannot, do for you.

 & This is why we publish a page with hundreds of real Online Trainer Academy students and include contact information for each. Legitimate education providers have nothing to hide and are proud to put you in touch with as many past students as you like. You can see our page at **theptdc.com/ota-stories.**

CHAPTER 5

Programming Fundamentals

How to Avoid the "Perfect" Workout Trap

"How do I get better at programming?"

That's probably the most common question I get from new trainers. The obvious answer would be to tell you how to get better at programming, but that wouldn't solve the real problem, which isn't a lack of programming skill but a lack of confidence. New trainers often worry about creating the "perfect" workouts for their clients. That's a classic trap.

Learning how to program is a lifelong journey. Every six months you should look back and be embarrassed at how you used to program six months ago. Accept it: You're never going to be able to create the perfect workout for your client, and you'll always be embarrassed by your past programming. "Best" doesn't exist. "Better" does, however, and you can always get better.

My goal with this chapter isn't to teach you about programming. That's for a later chapter. For now, my goal is threefold:

1. Give you the confidence to know that your programming at any given moment is probably good enough.
2. Help you recognize that a program is only as good as your ability to get a client to adhere to it.
3. Identify the common pitfalls inexperienced coaches encounter so you recognize when you're falling into a trap and can pull yourself out.

Other trainers are not laughing at you: get past imposter syndrome

As the new trainer at a gym, it may feel like all of the more experienced pros are judging your every move. They aren't.

All of us, at times, feel like frauds. This is "imposter syndrome." [⚭] If you've ever worried that one day you'll be exposed, you're not alone. New and experienced trainers battle it constantly.

Even if you sometimes feel like "that clueless trainer," take solace in knowing that the other trainers who work with you feel the same lack of confidence. These are the

---

⚭ *Here's a fantastic video on the "imposter syndrome" phenomenon:* **theptdc.com/imposter**.

sorts of quiescent thoughts that nobody discusses in the open and can lead a new trainer to believe that he or she is simply not good enough.

Personal training, particularly the program design aspect, is a mastery profession. There is no way to measure "best" and a client could be happy and get good results from countless different programs, whether you trained him or not. Who's to say that one program is better than another? How would you ever know? This, combined with the inflated egos in our industry, make it difficult for new trainers.

So let's talk about ego for a moment. Helping people get healthy, avoid disease, and love their bodies is important work that requires an ego. All good trainers have egos.

Below is my damaging admission. My hope is that by reading it you realize you're not alone. Everybody, even people like me who write books about this stuff, feels the way you do, and I hope knowing that gives you an ego boost.

My confession: We're all making it up.

We make good guesses, and those of us who truly care always strive to get better. Personal training requires mastery, where every trainer acts on hunches and works hard to figure out what works for coaching, physiology, and biomechanics. We hope we hit the right buttons to help our clients get results, and most of the time it works. But basically, we all make things up as we go.

I confess these things in the hopes that you gain the confidence to push forward and strive for mastery. That's the best you and any of us can do. If you're always getting better, you'll be one step ahead. You'll be awesome.

Some more truth

Let's break down how the "good enough" workout argument really works. Most of your clients will fall into the beginner-to-intermediate stage. (What I'm about to say does not apply to advanced clientele or competitive athletes). That means...

—Your beginner and intermediate clients will adapt well to countless stimuli. One workout you give them may be a bit better or a bit worse than another workout.

—You won't know if a workout is better or worse because the difference in the clients' short-term results will be negligible.

—Long-term results are what matter because those can be measured accurately.

—Long-term results achieved by "good enough" workouts performed consistently over time are the mark of a great trainer.

I recognize that this may sound like blasphemy and fly in the face of everything you've learned to date, but the truth is that there are probably a thousand programs that will work for your client. A "good enough" workout will do, as long as your client puts in the work. The importance of whether or not a program that you design is awesome pales in comparison to your ability to get a client to *want* to do that program.

Helping clients develop exercise adherence (a.k.a get 'em to *want* to work out)

It sounds weird to say, but you need to play with your clients' brains to get them thinking in a productive way. Adherence is largely dependent on self-efficacy, or the belief that one can achieve. If clients believe a program is right for them, it'll work. If they trust you, the odds of adherence, and, as a result, achievement, skyrocket.

This all makes sense ... in theory. In practice, it's a little more difficult. Telling a client that the program you designed for him is "good enough" doesn't instill confidence.

Imagine that you're talking to Jim about signing up. Jim is on the fence. You want to be honest with Jim, so you say:

"Hey, Jim, there are a bunch of different things that you could probably do to meet your goal of looking better in a T-shirt by adding a bit of muscle to your shoulders, arms, and upper back. The programming is quite basic, really. There's nothing special about what I'm doing.

What I'll give you is going to be good enough.
That cool?"

Although you're telling the truth, the odds that Jim hands over his credit card and eagerly attends every session are slim. To get him to buy the training and buy into the programming, Jim needs to believe that the program is perfect *for him*. [✐]

There isn't a straightforward solution to this problem, unfortunately. To navigate it, you need to learn how to be an amazing listener.

Be mindful of clients' earlier negative experiences

Years back, I had a client, Beth, who had worked with both a trainer (for eight months) and a circuit exercise instructor (for six months) before she came to me. She got lousy results with both.

Beth was over-busy. Her husband was fighting cancer and her grown kids were in the process of moving away. She worked full-time and wanted to lose some fat but couldn't. She pushed herself, ate enough of the right things (as far as I could tell), and stayed consistent. She should have been getting good results, but the weight wouldn't come off.

The problem, to me, seemed stress-induced. The

✐ *While the best fitness programs are usually the simplest, they require a sort of demented theatre to sell. More on this demented theatre here:* **onlinetrainer.com/theatre**.

other trainer and the circuit class gave her "metabolic workouts" involving lots of big muscle movements with light weights and really short breaks. Workouts like this give you a lot of total work, but I thought Beth just wasn't recovering like she should. Her body was worn down, so her stress response was through the roof, which kept the fat on. I suspected Beth had also lost confidence in her ability to reach her goal of losing fat.

I suggested that we do something totally different: train like a powerlifter. "I don't want you doing as much total work as you've been doing," I said, explaining the stress response and how it may be interfering with fat loss.**

Over the coming months, I trained her as a powerlifter. We did a much longer warm-up, a much longer cool-down, and far fewer reps (maybe 30 to 50) per workout. She started losing weight while learning how to lift a ton of it.

What happened next is much more interesting than any program or weight loss could ever be. Over time it became clear, after listening deeply to Beth, what her true goal really was. She didn't want to fit into a dress or look a certain way for an event or anything like that. She didn't even want to lose fat. Deep down, she wanted to have some control over something in her life because so much of her life was out of her control.

** *Who knows for sure if this is what was happening. When I spoke to Beth about my theory, I made sure that she knew it was just that: a theory. The body is so complex that we never really know. Since nothing else had worked, however, my theory made sense and was worth a shot.*

Her husband was dying. (He ended up passing away over the course of our training.) Her son was prepping to join the Israeli military. Her daughter had already moved away. She worked at a job with very little control over what she was doing. In fact, her entire life felt out of control.

After we changed her program, everything changed. Beth could now walk into the gym and crank a 200-pound deadlift. That made her feel great. She started sleeping better. She slowly became a happier, more confident person, and the weight just evaporated as a result.* And I had a client, and friend, for life.

Let's talk about listening

Listening — really listening — is a valuable skill. A client will tell you everything you ever need as long as you know how to ask the right questions and are patient enough to listen for the answers.

When you want to listen to a client, set the scene by removing distractions. Invite him into an office, close the door, and establish a power position — in other words, sit behind your desk while the client sits in a chair across from you. This sets up a dynamic where

---

* Maybe the fat loss was a result of her training more consistently because she loved it, or better at-home eating habits because she felt better about herself, or an improved hormonal balance due to a decrease in stress. Or all of the above. Or none of them. I don't know why what I did worked. But it did, and that's what matters. And that's the lesson. We can post-rationalize as much as we want, but at the end of the day we'll never really know. All we can do is make our best educated guesses and keep trying until something works.

the client is there to speak and you're there to help. It may take some time and be a bit of a struggle for him to open up about the real reason he's there.

Once you sit down, follow this conversation template:

First, engage. Find something unique about that person as an icebreaker. Unusual shoes, a unique piece of jewelry, a Hard Rock Mexico shirt. Anything. "Were you in Mexico?" or "That's a beautiful necklace. Is there a story behind it?"

Doing this builds a rapport. At the same time, try to mimic the person's actions. If he leans forward, so do you. If he speaks softly, so do you.

Next, transition. After this initial bout of rapport-building, move the conversation into why he's there. Your first question is easy: "So Jim, what's your fitness goal?"

Wait for a response, listen to the entire answer and, when he's done speaking, count to two before asking your next question that digs deeper into his goal. In an effective sales/goal-setting meeting, you always want to be the one asking the questions. If he answers with a question, respond back with a question. If you get stuck answering his questions, the power differential in the room shifts, and it becomes difficult to get the information you need to properly help the client.

Let's say you're talking with Jim. You ask, "What do you want to achieve?" and he says something that ends with, "Well, why should I choose you?" Then you'd say, "I don't know yet. First I need to know what it is that you want to achieve. What are you looking for?" Be cool, be polite, keep asking questions.

I mentioned earlier that you want to remain quiet for a few seconds after he's finished speaking. The reason is that he may not be done speaking yet, and silence makes things awkward. You *want* awkward.* When you're in a power position, and it's quiet in the room, it's the client's turn to talk. When people are in control, they have their barriers up and won't tell you what you really need to know. Make it awkward and you'll create a power differential where it's assumed it's Jim's turn to speak. This unease will make him more likely to keep talking and be honest. This is where he'll tell you the real reason why he's sitting across from you.

The first thing that most clients will say in a goal-setting meeting is something like, "I want to lose 20 pounds," but this information is pretty useless to you. A 20-pound weight loss is a meaningless goal unless it is placed in the proper context. Logic doesn't drive action. Emotion drives action. Logic justifies it.

In this situation, a logical goal like, "I want to lose 20 pounds" or "I want to get in better shape" or "I want to run a 5K" requires you to dig deeper. Saying something like, "Okay. How would losing weight make you feel?"

---

* *Make it as awkward in the room as it must've been when Luke Skywalker found out that Leia was his sister. (I made a promise years back that I would use this joke in every book I wrote. It's in the footnotes but still counts. So I guess this is a win).*

works. Your goal is to get a situation or story from Jim that will clue you in on the real, emotional reason he's exercising.

I worked with a woman named Kim early on in my training career (and no, not all clients' names rhyme; Jim is hypothetical, Kim is not). She wasn't having much success. That was my fault. I'd made the mistake of failing to get into the emotional reasons for exercising before we started training. A month or two in, she'd lost a bit of weight but wasn't happy with the results. I took her into my office, closed the door, and talked to her about why she wanted to exercise.

After some awkwardness, she admitted she had a memory of wearing this beautiful red flowing dress while on a cruise with her husband in the Bahamas. She said, "When I walked in the room, I felt like every woman was looking at me with jealousy, and I felt like every man was looking at me like they were jealous of my husband."

I had it. That was her reason for being there. *Red dress*. I could use that as her trigger.

The workout stayed the same, but how I communicated it drastically changed. My program, the exact same program as before, wasn't a workout with the goal of helping her lose 10 pounds, her original goal. It was a program to help her fit back into the red dress that she wore on the cruise with her husband. I changed the name of the program to "The Red Dress Experiment

— Day 1" instead of "Weight Loss Workout — Day 1."

When explaining the exercises, I sold her on them based on her *real* reason for being there. I'd say, "Okay, we're going to do goblet squats because they hammer the legs, where you have a lot of big muscles. Doing this causes a larger fat-loss response to help you get back into that red dress."

Same program. Same exercises. Same physiological function. Improved adherence.

The formula for getting your clients to adhere to exercise is quite basic:

Emotion drives action; logic justifies it.

Connecting goals and emotions differentiates you from free information online

Connecting your client's goal to an emotion helps develop adherence, but for some reason goal-setting isn't taught this way. More commonly, you're shown how to create quantitative goals (like "I want to lose 10 pounds") for your clients without connecting them to anything meaningful. That adherence to conventional programming, even with a personal trainer, is low, and it's no surprise.

There's a ton of free workout information online. A lot of people think, why pay when I don't have to? They'll have that basic goal in mind, lose 10 pounds, run a 5K charity race, or pack on muscle. So how do you separate yourself from ubiquitous free material? Connect your client's goal with his or her emotional reason. When it's personal like that, it can't be replicated in a book or online.

I'm quite familiar with the bookselling business and the personal training business. They're drastically different despite promoting common goals. Buying a fitness book is addictive. The thought that you're going to achieve whatever the book promises gives you a hit of "feel-good" dopamine. The more you believe you can achieve the promised goal, the bigger the hit.

People who buy fitness books rarely buy just one. This is a good thing for publishers. But if a fitness book's purpose is to get you in shape, why do people buy multiple books? Because the act of buying a book and dreaming about the changes it will bring is easy and feels good. The act of sticking to the program is hard and feels terrible.*

This is why goals are sold as "quick" and "easy" with "rock-hard results in just seven days." That hit of dopamine is addictive. It makes people want to get another hit, and another, and another, and another. This is why some people buy fitness book after fitness book yet never make any progress. By regularly publishing new titles, book publishers make it easy for you to get that hit of dopamine, and then you crave it and buy another book, and another, ad infinitum.

For most. Maybe you love working out, but most people would think that you're a little nutty in the head because, for them, it's miserable.

I never used to understand why people buy more than one fitness book until this concept became clear. By its very nature, the publishing industry profits when it sells more books, and the personal training business profits when it changes lives.

This is where you come in. You need to make the programs emotional to your clients. Find out their emotional goals, and relate everything you do back to those goals. Your clients will believe that their workouts are perfect for them, adherence will follow, and the odds of a positive, and life-changing, physical transformation increase.

WHEN A CLIENT ASKS ABOUT THE LATEST CELEBRITY WORKOUT

So your client comes in convinced that the latest celebrity fitness fad is magical, then asks to change course even though they're already making good progress on your program. How do you handle it?

My client Brittany came in with a magazine one day with an article about the Tracy Anderson Workout. (Tracy Anderson is a celebrity trainer who believes that women should not lift more than three pounds at a time while doing hundreds of reps). Anderson has worked with celebrities including Gwyneth Paltrow (who's an investor in Anderson's company), and her workout garnered a lot of media attention at the time.

My client questioned why we were lifting heavy weights, and said, "I want to pull my skin closer to my muscles. That's what her workout does." And no joke, the popular magazine said that doing extremely high reps of low-weight exercises for women can pull the skin closer to the muscle.

Now, you can't pull skin close to muscle. I'm pretty sure that's physiologically impossible. But I hadn't done a good enough job of making Brittany emotionally engaged in her workout, so she was distracted by the latest fad. I tried to convince her that the claims made by a popular magazine were wrong, but failed. I ended up losing that client.

If I'd connected my programming to my client's real, emotional goal at the start and revisited that goal throughout, I never would've been in that situation. Once a client comes in with a magazine or quotes an authority questioning your programming, you're in deep, and it's going to be hard to recover. In my case, it was my word against the word of the magazine and celebrities that Brittany admired. There was nothing I *could've said or done to win that fight.*

Your only chance is to make it known to your client that the workout you prepared was done for them, and only them, and that it will take them to where they really want to go.

THE TAKEAWAY

Your ability to make clients *want* to do their workouts is more important than what's in the workouts.

CHAPTER 6

Keep It Simple
A Workout Programming Strategy

Your cert likely gave you an introduction to programming. My goal with this chapter is to simplify the act of programming, give you the steps to build on your knowledge, and teach you how to sell your programs to clients. As you already learned, a program is only as good as your ability to get a client to *want* to do it.

Programming can (and probably should) be simple

While your skill in developing programs will evolve over time, the better your system for writing them, the easier time you'll have. The first step for building a client's program is to identify his or her goals, which we talked about. Then, when it's time to write the nuts and bolts, your starting point is the rep range.

Rep range is the great decider. Once you identify it, everything in the program follows. There's nothing fancy about rep ranges. You probably learned them as part of your certification. The basics are all you need to know. While there is some variation, the rep ranges are:

- 1 to 5 reps — Strength/power
- 6 to 10 reps — Hypertrophy
- 11 to 15+ reps — Endurance/fat loss[*]

Step one: Choose the ideal rep range for the client's main exercises, the ones you'll use as the baseline for her progression. This should align with her overall goals.

Step two: Choose two to four appropriate main exercises for the client based on the rep range. A lower rep range generally dictates a more energy-intensive exercise. Most common are large, multi-joint movements: squats, deadlifts, or Olympic lifts. As you increase the number of reps, the exercise selection could change to movements that are less form-intensive and therefore won't suffer from increased volume.

Step three: Determine the number of sets, tempo, and rest intervals. All of these programming considerations follow the rep range. Here's an overview. (Note: There can be a lot more variation and nuance, but this is good enough for now).

---

[*] This doesn't mean you don't burn fat when working at 6 reps or that power development is impossible at 11 reps. There is crossover at all levels.

1 TO 5 REPS — STRENGTH/POWER

- # of sets: A lot. Anywhere from 3 to 10.
- Tempo**: Explosive. 10X0 or similar.

REST INTERVAL: COMPLETE. 3 TO 5 MINUTES.

- 6 to 10 reps — Hypertrophy
- # of sets: Varies. Usually 2 to 4.
- Tempo: Long. 4020 or similar.
- Rest interval: Incomplete. 1 to 1.5 minutes.

11 TO 15+ REPS — ENDURANCE/FAT LOSS

- # of sets: Varies. Usually 1 to 3 circuits.
- Tempo: Not considered.
- Rest interval: Incomplete. 0 to 1 minute.

The number of days a week that the client trains will depend on the desired training stimulus that you want to elicit, but you must also consider the realities of your client's schedule. You should have already discussed how often a client is realistically willing and able to train.

Experienced programmers will tell you that as they learn more, they build simpler programs and rely on the basics. For most clients, nothing fancy is necessary. Figure out what they want to achieve, identify the number of reps, and let the rest of the pieces fall into place naturally.

** *Tempo is traditionally denoted as four numbers each corresponding to different parts of the lift in seconds. It goes eccentric — pause — concentric — pause. So in the case of a bench press that starts with the barbell racked, the first number is the amount of time you take to bring the bar to your chest. The second number is the pause with the bar on your chest. The third number is the time you take to press the bar back up (X means as explosive as possible). The fourth number is the time paused before repeating the entire thing again.*

Step four: Choose secondary exercises to fill in the bulk of the program. These movements support the primary movements, and can include pretty much anything but are usually limited to less energy-intensive movements. Single-joint exercises, weak-point training, and high-intensity cardio exercises like sled pushes or weighted carries can all fit in here. The secondary exercises fill in the gaps and are important, but progress is measured by your primary exercises.

Step five (if applicable): Add in tertiary exercises at the end. These are commonly referred to as prehabilitation movements ("prehab"). With prehab, consider places where your client may be susceptible to injury based on existing imbalances, lifestyle habits, or previous injuries. Choose exercises that help reduce the risk of injury.*

In another, and more personal, example, I have transitioned from a very active lifestyle as a personal trainer to a reasonably sedentary life, one where I work out at a predetermined time and then spend the rest of my day working out my phalanges, sitting and writing. I want to ensure that I can write books for many more years. Desk ergonomics and taking care of my wrists, elbows, and forearms are important. My personal prehab includes soft tissue work on my forearms and

---

* For example, somebody who loves to ride her bike for long distances probably has strong legs but a sore back. In addition to getting stronger overall, this person would benefit from some glute, adductor, and upper-back work. Probably.

radial deviation work** to offset the demands of typing.

Improve your programming

What I just covered is a simplified programming approach. Now it's time to talk about getting better at the science, and art, of it. It's a nuanced thing to learn and hard to teach. I can't show you programming for every client you might encounter. I prefer to show you how to find the best resources and what to do with them moving forward.

Programming how-to books exist for trainers. You'd do well to read a few, but they can be pretty dry, and much of what I've seen is geared towards high performance, not the everyday client.

Early in my career, a manager of mine tried to improve the programming skills of all staff trainers. She'd meet with every trainer once a week to review our clients' programs. She also wanted us to create three-month periodized training plans for each client.

At that point, I didn't know much about periodization. I did the obvious thing and bought a bunch of textbooks on it, including one by a strength coach named Tudor Bompa. (This wasn't the only one, just the name that I remember.)

** *Picture yourself with your arm straight ahead of you with thumb pointing up holding a light bar (works well with straight bar handle attachments for the cable machine). Pull your thumb up toward the inside of your elbow, focusing on using the musculature on the radial side of your posterior forearm.*

Bompa's text blew my mind. Geez, programming was complex! This book covered programming for high performance across multiple sports and included everything from off-season, to in-season, to tapering, to recovering from injuries, and everything in between. My eyes bled as I flipped the pages, trying to make sense of it, all the while freaking and thinking, *If I don't know all of this, I'm a terrible trainer and a failure and everybody will laugh at me and maybe I should just go get a job with a desk.*

Wanting to make a good impression in my weekly meeting with the manager, I built complicated, periodized programs for my clients. I thought that they were programming poetry, but looking back, they were pretty terrible for one obvious reason:

> *Clients hardly ever finished them.*

Heavily periodized programs are built for people who plan their lives around fitness and performance. Our clients are the opposite. We're here to help fit fitness into their lives.*

It became so rare for a client to follow the complete program, with no interruptions, that I stopped programming far in advance. Clients got sick. Their kids got sick. They forgot about a workout, or had an unexpected work trip. *Something* would get in the way. We're dealing with real people living real lives.

---

* *A trainer's goal is to remove stress from a client's life, not add to it. Never forget that.*

This experience showed me in no uncertain terms that much of the mind-numbingly complex material in these programming books could never apply to a conventional personal training client. Granted, these textbooks can give you some ideas, but there are usually better, simpler ways.

Another way to improve your programming is to discuss your current programs with the local trainer mastermind group that I advised you to form earlier in this book.

A third way to improve: Read books and other materials aimed at consumers, not trainers. If you have a specific clientele you want to train, buy and study books, videos, courses, and online programs aimed at that population. Deconstructing these programs will teach you more than any technical book on programming ever will.

Let's say you train two different client types: women whose primary goal is fat loss, and female athletes. Buy all the books and programs you can find that deal with those types of clients. First, anything that is mass-marketed to consumers, or "consumer-facing," is going to be much cheaper than professional development, or quote/unquote "certifications." A book may cost you $20 to $50 while a certification course will cost you hundreds or even thousands. This cost comes down to the "value proposition" that the person producing a certification course is able to make.

WHAT'S A VALUE PROPOSITION ("VALUE PROP")?

A value prop is how much money you stand to make as a result of some information — and your justification for making the move (or not). I could justifiably argue that $500 is a fair price for an online course because, if you charge $50/hour, then the information contained within the course needs to get you 10 client hours via retention or referrals to pay for itself. Depending on the information, I could also argue that the course will teach you some new skills, which means you'll be able to access a new group of clients. That'll be worth a certain amount of money, as well.

Value propositions are important to understand when selling your program, as they help you justify the cost of your training. Let's say, for example, you're selling a 12-week package to golfers to improve mobility and increase strength. Your value prop: Tell them they could buy that new expensive driver for $1,000, or go through your training for only $500 and hit the ball just as far.

If you can't sell a program, it doesn't matter how good you are at making it. Crafting appropriate and persuasive value propositions helps.

Tap other sources to get your client's buy-in

Mass-market materials geared toward consumers contain a ton of information that can help you sell your programs (and usually build them, as well). Let's say you have marathoner clients, so you buy a book aimed at female runners. The book includes training plans, plus the explanations for them and why specific exercises are included. You already learned how to study this information, but the secret sauce is in the book's language. It may be the perfect type of language to use to connect with your clients.

Read these books, study the "trigger" words they use, review the cues, and write down phrases from exercise descriptions. How do they express the benefits of a squat versus how you describe it in the gym?

Highlight useful phrases so that you can use them to describe your programming to improve the buy-in from clients. As you've learned, talking to your clients about the programs you've developed and getting them excited about jumping in are almost as important as the programs themselves.

You may recall that I told you not to rely solely on material your clients may read. And you shouldn't. If you're reading widely, you'll be absorbing information from many sources. Use these mass-market materials as idea generators. When you get a good idea or find something interesting, you can take a step back, do a little more of your own research, and see whether you can apply this idea to your own program.

Yes, you should create program templates

Every great trainer I know uses templates to some extent. There's nothing wrong with templates. Why continually reinvent the wheel? If you've done the work to create the best program possible for a specific type of client and another individual comes in with similar needs, why start from scratch? But wait, doesn't that, by definition, mean that the next client won't get your best possible workout?

I don't want you to misunderstand me — you're not giving the same program to different clients. Instead, you've found a formula that works, have a template as a foundation, and can individualize it according to each client's needs, assessments, and any other variables. As you learn more about programming, your templates improve.

I suggest you make one program template for every type of client you work with. A 30- to 40-year-old professional male who trains three times a week and sits at a desk for his job will have a different template than a new mom. Each client can be placed into a reasonably broad category, so if you create a sensible number of templates across several categories, you should have an obvious place to start with each newbie.

The Template in Practice: A Totally-Hypothetical-But-Incredibly-Useful Case Study

THE CLIENT CATEGORY:
20- to 30-year-old men who are slim, generally healthy, and have been training for at least a year with unsatisfactory results. These men have no major injuries and want to put on 10 to 15 pounds of muscle.

Here's my made-up template[*] for one day of programming:

Exercise 1:
Barbell front squat — 4 sets. 6 to 8 reps. 4020 tempo. 1.5 min rest

Exercise 2a:
Bench press — 3 sets. 6 to 8 reps. 4020 tempo

Exercise 2b:
DB lateral raise — 3 sets. 12 to 15 reps. 2010 tempo. 1.5 min rest

Exercise 3a:
Barbell bent-over row (t-bar, landmine, or barbell) — 3 sets. 6 to 8 reps. 4020 tempo

Exercise 3b:
Goblet squat — 3 sets. 12 to 15 reps. 2010 tempo. 1.5 min rest

---

* This is just an example. Whether you agree with my programming or not is irrelevant. Instead, review it while reading the next section to understand how templating works in action.

Exercise 4a:

Seated incline DB biceps curl (supinated grip) — 4 sets. 10 to 12 reps. 4010 tempo

Exercise 4b:

Standing DB biceps curl (supinated grip) — 4 sets. 10 to 12 reps. 4010 tempo

Exercise 4c:

Standing DB biceps curl (neutral grip) — 4 sets. 10 to 12 reps. 4010 tempo. 1.5 min rest[*]

Using my workout as a template, let's say you have a client who experiences some shoulder pain while bench pressing. No problem. It could be smaller-than-optimal space in his acetabulum, an impingement, some sort of inflammation, or just a bad day because he slept on it funny. You're not a doctor, so you don't really know. If you're worried, you should refer him to a physiotherapist. But if you're not worried, then you can easily adapt the template to avoid exercise 2a, the bench press.

In this example, an easy way to alleviate the strain in the shoulder is to do an incline dumbbell neutral-grip press. Instead of being locked into a position with a barbell, neutral-grip dumbbells give the shoulder joint more freedom. The exercise would still be done at the

---

And when you get to this point in the workout you can smile at you client and say that it's arm-agedden time.
No? Nothing? Not even a smile? Okay, I'll keep trying. How about, "Come one, come all, and get your two tickets to the gun show?"

same point in the workout for three sets, six to eight reps, and a 4020 tempo.

Templates are most commonly individualized with progressions, regressions, and workarounds for exercises. The placement in the program, sets, reps, tempo, and rest stay consistent and almost never change between clients with similar goals.

THE TAKEAWAY

Keep your programming simple. Creating workout templates will save you time and still allow you to customize workouts for clients.

CHAPTER 7

Avoid the Hype
Why Fitness Trends Are Traps

Hang around the industry long enough and you can spot the latest fad a mile away. The fitness industry is like a pendulum swinging back and forth. Everything new and amazing has already come and gone. To illustrate, here's a quick history lesson.

Set the time machine for 1951

The Jack LaLanne Show first aired in 1951, and lasted 34 years. The athletic, muscular, and charismatic LaLanne did everything he could to make exercise appealing and accessible to anyone who might be watching, from kids to grandparents. (He lived to be 96, so even back then he was on to something).

In 1968, Kenneth Cooper published *Aerobics*, a book that presented endurance training as the only worthwhile form of exercise. He dismissed what he called "muscular fitness" as "putting a lovely new coat of paint on an automobile that really needs an engine overhaul."

The "aerobics" craze lasted decades. Judi Sheppard Missett introduced Jazzercise in 1969. *Jane Fonda's Workout*, released in 1982, became the bestselling VHS tape in history at the time. Richard Simmons released *Sweatin' to the Oldies* in 1998. Spandex leotards became a thing.

Jonathan Goldberg, a personal trainer from South Africa who'd reinvented himself as an endurance cyclist named Johnny G, also reinvented indoor group exercise when he introduced Spinning in 1994. Never mind that stationary bikes had already been around for decades. Bike shorts are now standard gym attire.

All this time, the pendulum swung back and forth between high and low intensity. While the '90s gave us Tae Bo, Pilates, Curves, and Zumba, the 2000s gave us P90X and CrossFit. Throwing up at the gym became a point of pride.

The 2000s also gave us "functional" training with balls: Swiss, medicine, Bosu. Don't forget the TRX, too. In the 2010s it's been more of the same: Insanity and Tracy Anderson, Orangetheory Fitness and Planet Fitness, and everything in between.

There's always something new, and it's usually based on what promoters decide is the "most important aspect of fitness," whether that's heart-rate range or mobility or metabolic fitness or Olympic lifts.

Then there are the diets. Every five to 10 years, some new low-carb variation blows up and marketers go crazy for it. Atkins, South Beach, Paleo, Bulletproof, keto. They're all easy to sell because, for those who can stick to them, weight loss is pretty much automatic, a neat side effect of nixing the biggest carb source: highly processed foods.

And I haven't even mentioned the completely made-up stuff like detoxes and cleanses and spot reduction. You get the picture.

Nothing appeals to everyone

Now, it's easy to dump on fads. If there's a lesson here, it's that lots of fads can coexist. The 1970s gave us bodybuilding legends pumping iron at Gold's Gym in Venice Beach. But just a few miles away, in Beverly Hills, Richard Simmons opened a gym for overweight people who didn't feel welcome at traditional health clubs. For every craze that interests millions, many millions more are interested in something completely different.

And yet, for all the attention given to those fads, a huge percentage of the population is still sedentary. The fitness movements popular at any given moment simply don't appeal to as many people as we imagine. And even those who get into them eventually become distracted or bored, and either move on or relapse into inactivity.

People respond to different stimuli in different ways. For example, some people want to work with a trainer one-on-one. We all know this, of course; it's how our profession got started. But for others, it's a miserable experience. Work one-on-one with a stranger? In a place where you aren't comfortable to begin with? Not happening.

Some people love group exercise; some don't. Some people like the Curves model, where they follow a prescribed circuit workout at a gym. Others seek out new programs in magazines, videos, or books.

Online training appeals to a lot of people, in part because they aren't limited to a trainer down the street. They can do their own research and find the person they think is best, even if he or she happens to be on the other side of the world. Others need the accountability of a coach beside them.

Meanwhile, the majority of people who work out don't want any guidance at all. They're happy to do what they enjoy and what works for them without someone telling them what to do or how to do it. That doesn't mean they won't respond to a new option that comes along. In many ways, we as an industry are just getting started.

That's the first insight from this little history lesson: Fads come and go. They always have. They always will. Some pendulum swings are more extreme than others, but the repeating pattern is always the same.

The second insight: You never have to worry about

missing out on a fad because of the one thing that *doesn't* change.

The pendulum always swings back

Human physiology isn't static, of course. We continue to evolve, responding to changes in our environment, food chain, and lifestyle. But if you look only at the past few hundred years, we've stayed pretty much the same.

Here's the craziest part: Not only has our physiology stayed the same, but for well over 100 years we've also known what type of fitness is necessary for health, vitality, and appearance.

Chad Landers, the founder of Push Private Fitness in L.A., is an avid collector of old fitness books. His bookshelf is a museum of ancient (to us) texts and long-lost methods. When staying at his house, I leafed through some of the books in his collection.

One tattered green book caught my eye: *How to Get Strong and How to Stay So*. It was written in 1879 — yes, 1879 — by William Blaikie. (With a Google search, you can find and download a free digital version.)

The book begins:

> *Probably more men walk past the corner of Broadway and Fulton Street, in New York City, in the course of one year, than any other point in America. Men of all nations and ages, heights and weights. Look at them carefully as they pass, and*

you will see that scarcely one in ten is ... thoroughly well-built. Some slouch their shoulders and double in at the waist; ... this one has one shoulder higher than the other and that one both too high; some have heavy bodies and light legs; others the reverse; and so on, each with his own peculiarities. A thoroughly... well-proportioned man, easy and graceful in his movements, is far from a frequent sight.

Yes, even in 1879, a fitness book talked about the importance of posture and proportioned physiques. And the author was talking about it not just from an aesthetic point of view, but in terms of health. This was long before anyone talked about cars and computers distorting our posture and making us more sedentary. (Although, coincidentally, the first automobile patent was filed in 1879).

But wait, there's more!

Blaikie also made an argument for young women to take up resistance training:

Observe the girls in and of our cities or towns, as they pass to and from school, and see how few of them are at once blooming, shapely, and strong ... Instead of high chests, plump arms, comely figures, and a graceful and handsome mien,* you constantly see flat chests, angular shoulders, often round and warped forward, with scrawny necks, pipe-stem arms, narrow backs, and a weak walk.

---

* *The word "mien" really needs to be used more.*

Today we all agree on the importance of women's health, athleticism, and strength. But Blaikie wrote about it more than 100 years before Bev Francis squared off with Rachel McLish in *Pumping Iron II: The Women*.

If you read through the entire book and update the language to contemporary English, you'll see workout advice that's similar to what we recommend today.

But here's the dilemma: Even if you understand that very little is new, how do you sell something old? You really can't. That's why the pendulum has been swinging for well over 100 years. We go crazy for crazes, only to realize that the craze is either too intense, too easy, too boring, or too much of something else. Maybe one day we wake up and say, "These leotards look ridiculous. What was I thinking?" But then we pick up some neon short-shorts, and we're off to the next big thing.

My advice? Don't pay attention to crazes or fads. Do what you do with your programming and coaching, and learn to sell its proven benefits. That's how you build a successful career. Attempting to keep up with the next big thing is the best way to ensure you're always one step behind. Even if you manage to catch the wave at just the right moment and get out ahead of your peers, it's just a matter of time before something else comes along and you're scrambling to catch up. Base your business on a fad, and you're doomed when that fad disappears — along with your clients.

It's okay to be interested in new things, and even to experiment with them, especially when they excite your clients. Just make sure you aren't taken in or taken over by those new things.

Clever marketers make it sound like they've discovered something genuinely groundbreaking. Or uncovered some ancient secret, or found a way to hack human physiology. They haven't. It's all just a rehash of something that came before. There's nothing like reading a fitness book from 1879 to drive that point home.

THE TAKEAWAY

Fitness trends come and go, but the fundamentals never go out of style.

CHAPTER 8

Polish Your Reputation

Get Clients to Ask You to Train Them

About three years into my career, I started training a client who would soon become my greatest mentor. He passed along my (now famous) two golden rules, which I'm honored to pass along to you. I have followed these rules every day since, and they've guided me the whole way.

The Two Golden Rules

The first rule: **Do a great job.**

The second rule: **Make sure everybody knows about it.**

It sounds simple, and it is. But this is the secret to getting more clients, not just today, but deep into the future. If you're not already doing a great job, that's your priority. Once you are confident enough in your work, then it's time to develop skills that'll make people aware of just how good and passionate and knowledgeable you are.

There's no single way to magically create a line of clients begging you to train. This happens over time as you work to establish a reputation that precedes you. If you haven't figured it out yet, reputation is *huge* in our industry. In this chapter, I'm going to highlight the major areas to develop to give you the best chance of being in the right place at the right time when a potential client is looking for a trainer. This way, when the client's ready, you're the only clear choice. She approaches you, wanting to train, without a sensitivity to price or comparing you to anybody else.

First things first: your elevator pitch

In less than 10 seconds, you need to be able to tell people exactly what you do, and how it will help them. Often referred to as an elevator pitch, this is your answer you give whenever somebody asks, "What do you do?"

I discourage replying with anything resembling, "I'm a personal trainer." That term has a pre-established meaning in many people's minds. Sometimes positive, sometimes negative, and always out of your control. Be different.

In fact, when someone asks, "What do you do?" you want your answer to not just be polite, but lead to business. Your answer should be specific enough so the person thinks of somebody who may be perfect for you. So dial in on who you train. You're new and may not have a good answer for this yet. That's okay. For now, you can be a bit less specific, but over time you'll want to get as specific as possible as you learn who your ideal client is.

Here are two examples of potential elevator pitches:

> *"I help guys feel more confident in a T-shirt by developing strong arms and burning unwanted stomach fat."*

Or:

> *"I help busy new moms focus on their health and fitness in the limited time they have so they feel as vital and energized as possible."*

Write your one- to two-sentence pitch and practice it.

Write Well: the successful trainer's secret weapon

Beyond your pitch, writing may be your most important tool. Keep it sharp. You don't have to be a word-processing maestro cranking out full articles or even a blog. But communicating yourself properly through the written word is critical. Something as simple as an email can make or break a client interaction.

For example, in the Online Trainer Academy (the certification I developed for trainers looking to take their services online, which you can learn more about at **theptdc.com/ota**), I show you how to build an online training program that includes sending strategic emails to clients. It's based on fun, psychological tricks, and works wonders without being sleazy or anything like that (sleazy always being a good thing to avoid, of course). When a coach who had invested in the program told me he wasn't getting the responses he should, I asked him to show me the emails he was sending to clients.

The problem was right there in black and white. Not only were the emails riddled with typos and grammatical errors, the messages were composed so poorly that they could've been written by a five-year-old.*

You could be saying the exact same thing as somebody else — even someone with inferior training chops — but if the other person articulates the what and the why better than you, they'll get the sale (and client).

Write well. This is the single most important tip I can give any new trainer who wants to differentiate him- or herself. Even something as simple as checking in with a client or potential lead, asking how his kids are, will make a better impression if well-written. Your message should be clear, easy to read, and (mostly) typo-free. Remember, your reputation is on the line.

---

* I now include done-for-you scripts in that section of the cert training.

Get the word out

You've got your elevator pitch. You've worked on your writing skills. The next step is to get some local media coverage to set you apart from other area trainers. While this coverage may get you some clients, the likelihood that it'll drive traffic and clientele to you is low. I recommend getting at least one piece of local media coverage early on because it acts as powerful trust and proof element when selling your service before you have a big book of client testimonials and transformations to promote.

To get the attention of the local media, you'll need a Twitter profile. If you already have one, then tweak it based on my suggestions and you're good to go. You don't need a lot of followers on Twitter to take advantage of its potential. Twitter isn't for content promotion; it's best used for connection. That's why we start there.

Your first step is to set up your profile properly. Upload a hi-res picture of your smiley face as your profile pic, not a logo. Your bio should say something about your fitness and health expertise. Your elevator pitch works well here. Finally, make sure that your location is set to your city. This is important when you reach out to local writers.

Now that your Twitter profile is up, figure out who's in charge of the "information network" in your neighborhood. Start with the media. There are probably several different papers and magazines that serve your area. Some local, some regional. Begin with the smaller, closer ones.

Pick up a copy of each publication and look through it (or, if it's online-only, you know what to do). When you see articles on health, fitness, or nutrition, find the byline. You can see who else works there on the masthead, which is found on the first few pages of the publication that lists the editorial staff.

Make a note of that writer's name and Twitter handle if he or she has one, and follow the corresponding account on Twitter. If the Twitter handle isn't mentioned in the publication (and it usually won't be), you'll have to do some digging. If a Twitter account exists for the person in question, it should be pretty easy to find with a bit of Googling (in fact, you may have to Google to find the online presence of the writer, as most these days are freelance).

Once you're following most of the reporters who cover health and fitness in your area, it's time to be patient, be supportive, and build relationships with them. Pop in there once every few days, read articles that they share, and try to respond intelligently. Retweet their work every so often. If you share a common interest (this doesn't have to be fitness), bring it up or send them an article you think they may enjoy. You don't have to respond to every single tweet. Instead, your goal is to stay at the top of their minds.

After a few interactions, this person will inevitably check out who the heck you are and voila! Guess what? You're a local fitness and health expert.

What many don't realize about the media is that reporters are constantly looking for reliable sources and good stories. After a while, they may approach you for quotes or to be a source for a story that they're working on.[*]

Even if they don't approach you for quotes, after a little bit of rapport-building back and forth — say a month or two — you can message them and say, "Hey, if you ever need anybody to talk about..." and list a couple of things you're an expert in, like fat loss or muscle growth. You may say, "If you ever need somebody for quotes, or a source for an article, or anything like that, I'm happy to help."[**]

Three Quick Ways People Will Perceive You as the Expert

According to Robert B. Cialdini, author of *Influence: The Psychology of Persuasion*, the three things that most contribute to the perception of expertise are title, clothing, and trappings.

---

[*] *I've even had trainers become sources for writers who later became clients. It's all business.*

[**] *I have no idea whether Twitter still exists as you're reading this. You don't have to use Twitter specifically. When I wrote this book, Twitter was the best option. What you're looking for is a platform most of your targeted people use, where they promote their stuff, where they likely have notifications turned on, and where there's little-to-no interaction.*

1. *Title*

Anybody can call himself a personal trainer. A lot of people with a lot less education and passion than you refer to themselves as personal trainers, so you're going to be lumped in with them unless you give yourself a better title.

In my book *Ignite the Fire*, I talk about a trainer named Roger Lawson, and how he calls himself "the Chief Sexification Officer." What a great title. I'd train with him. You can also call yourself a coach, or a fat-loss expert, or a new mom's motivator. Make it specific to what you do, and a little bit different.

2. *Clothing*

Dress the part. A good rule of thumb: Dress one step above the rest of your cohorts. If they're wearing sweatpants, you wear khakis. If they're wearing a dirty workout tee, wear a collared shirt. Immediately, you'll be perceived as more intelligent than they are.

Obviously, this is harder if your gym has a dress code. If so, make sure your clothes are wrinkle-free and your shoes clean, and you always look put-together.

3. *Trappings*

Trappings refer to your surroundings. You should always be around clients, and you should always be happy. The people in your orbit should be smiling, laughing, and jovial. Don't let onlookers at your club see you as bored, glum, or aloof.

I've walked into gyms all over the world and seen trainers sitting in their offices, with their feet up, on their cellphones, looking restless. They look like they have nothing to do. I don't want to train with them.

Even if you don't have a client, do your best to find a member to chat with on the floor. Get him or her in your office. Laugh together. Slap hands. Nobody wants to train with you if you aren't in demand, so always make it look like you are.

Do a great job and make sure everybody knows about it

If you follow my two golden rules and do the simple things listed in this chapter reliably and consistently, you'll quickly find yourself in demand, viewed as the expert, with clients seeking you out.

If you ignore the rules and use "tricks" to get clients, you'll find yourself in an endless cycle of client acquisition with no time or energy to train people. Oh, and word will get out about how you work. It always does.

THE TAKEAWAY

Reputation is everything in the fitness industry. Position yourself as an expert and make yourself visible, and potential clients will seek you out.

CHAPTER 9

Create Some Buzz
Four No-Fail Marketing Plans

In the fitness industry, you are the product. This is true for every trainer. Everybody lives by selling something, and you, my friend, get to sell the best thing there is: yourself.

I want you to be proud and confident of what you're selling. You should market, and when you find somebody who could benefit from your services, it's your responsibility to sell hard. No scheming required, and you don't have to resort to scummy, scammy, or slimy tricks. These are all misconceptions that scare too many good trainers away from marketing.*

Marketing sounds intimidating, but it simply comes down to figuring out what people want and, if

---

Early on, I too fell prey to the myth of the trainer who "just wants to help people," thinking that if I gave away my services for free or cheap, then I could help more. This myth is the exact opposite of what happens. Money needs to exchange hands for most people to take action, and it takes money to elicit large-scale change.

appropriate, positioning yourself and your skills as the go-to. If it's not appropriate, then it means being comfortable saying that you're not the right person to help.

In this chapter, I'll share four high-integrity marketing strategies. Some of them will get you clients overnight, but most involve playing the long game, putting the pieces in place for the future. You may be surprised how obvious some of what I'm going to tell you sounds. Don't underestimate it. The simple and obvious stuff is often the most important. And what young trainers almost always get wrong.

Marketing Method #1: Improve your day-to-day conversations

Told you that we're going back to basics! You already speak to people on a daily basis. Those people are potential clients, and everybody they know and interact with are potential clients. All you need to do is get them to like you and communicate what it is that you do and who you do it for. Sounds basic, but, as you read the following few paragraphs, you'll realize how important it is to have a strategy going into day-to-day conversations.

In social situations, the most common question is, "What do you do for a living?" It happens often, if not every day, and if you're at a party, multiple times.

You probably say something like "I'm, uhh, I'm a

personal trainer," and blabber on for a minute or two trying to fill the silence because that's what we do when we're uncomfortable and ill-prepared for a social situation.

Responding with your elevator pitch that you created earlier is an improvement, and not so bad. But we can do even better. Ideally, as you get more confident, you'll be able to save your elevator pitch for social media profiles and website "about" pages, where you don't have the advantage of a back-and-forth. But in conversation? It's your time to flourish.

Ask Questions: In almost all cases, a person only asks what you do to be polite. It's the socially accepted way to begin a conversation when there's nothing else to talk about. I want you to do what every great coach does: Ask questions.

The better way to respond is a variation of, "I help people achieve their fitness and health goals. Let's take you, for example. Do you have any fitness and health goals?" Now you are in the driver's seat. Now you've provided him the chance to speak about himself, given the conversation direction, and created an opportunity to find out what he's interested in. Usually, he'll tell you what he's trying to do fitness-wise, ask you questions about some trend, or say, "So you're a personal trainer?"

Sometimes they'll say that they don't have goals — in which case, congratulate them (never make someone feel bad for not having fitness goals), and work to build a rapport. Being a good conversationalist is an important skill for a trainer. Fortunately, it's relatively easy.

Your goal when having a conversation with somebody new is finding a point of mutual interest — a commonality. These classic conversation starters come from Dale Carnegie, author of *How to Win Friends and Influence People*:

1. What's your name?
2. Where do you live?
3. Do you have a family?
4. What do you do for a living?
5. Do you have any hobbies / sports?
6. Do you have any travel plans?

The questions, admittedly, are stiff and a little obvious. The secret is working them into a conversation naturally. When speaking with somebody new, they're feeling the awkwardness just as much as you are. As the conversation progresses, here's a list of things to keep in mind from Scott Adams, the creator of the comic *Dilbert*.

1. Ask questions.
2. Don't complain (much).
3. Don't talk about boring experiences (TV show, meal, dream, etc.)
4. Don't dominate the conversation. Let others talk.
5. Don't get stuck on a topic. Keep moving.
6. Planning is useful but it isn't conversation.
7. Keep the sad stories *short*, especially medical stories.

If you make the other person feel good, he'll like you. And if he likes you, he'll want to work with you and support you.

After your conversation, he may ask if you're looking for clients or ask to set up a meeting. If so, cool, set up a time. Usually he won't. You're not at a social gathering with the goal of converting clients. After a good conversation, ask if he wants to connect on Facebook. That, or say that you'd love to send him more info on whatever you spoke of, whether it's fat loss, shoulder pain, or whatever. Ask for the person's email so you can send that along. Follow up the next day via email with an article or blog post that you think he may be interested in based on your conversation.

Follow Up: When you follow up the next day, use your professional email account and set your email signature to have the name of your company (if you don't have a company name yet, just use your name followed by "Training"; so I'd be Jon Goodman Training), and your website (if you have one, which you should).

Keep following up with this person every few weeks just to say hi. The person may message you back after you send him that initial piece of information. He may not. You could send an article. You could send a study. As you come across more stuff that you find interesting, or think that the person may find interesting, pass it along. Or just say, "Hey, it was so great meeting you a couple of weeks ago. I just wanted to see how you're doing.

When you get a chance, I'd love to hear one thing that's going well with you."

That's one of my favorite ways to follow up with somebody. Ask someone, "What's one thing that's going awesome for you right now?" and you almost always get a response.

It's simple to take an everyday conversation and make yourself the go-to in fitness for that person, and that's really what it's all about. Whenever he, or maybe somebody that he knows, is ready for a trainer, you'll be top of mind.

A Real-Life Example: I was at my best friend's birthday party, chatting with an acquaintance. I didn't know him particularly well, but we'd crossed paths a couple of times, and he knew I was a trainer.

He told me that he'd worked with a trainer he believed had hurt him. He'd been doing fairly heavy deadlifts while standing on a Bosu ball and hurt his back. Whether it was the trainer's fault or not was irrelevant. This guy was hurt, and he could no longer ride his motorcycle or go mountain biking.

He hated not being able to enjoy his hobbies, which I realized was his emotional reason for wanting to get better. He had seen massage therapists and acupuncturists, and sometimes it would help a bit, but inevitably the pain would start again.

My new friend worked in construction. Recovery

methods like acupuncture and massage therapy are great, but not by themselves, especially if the problem is aggravated the next day. He either had an injury to be dealt with or needed some serious strengthening in addition to the recovery.

After listening to his story, I told him a little bit about low-back rehab and the importance of strengthening his back and glutes, not just treating the symptoms with things like massage therapy and acupuncture. I said strengthening, combined with those things, would be great for his back.

I discovered that he was doing what a lot of people do when they have low-back pain: stretching the hamstrings. The hamstrings often get tight to protect the back when it's unstable. Stretching the hamstrings won't help and could make things worse.

Anyway, this conversation went on for a while. I asked for his email at the end of our conversation and said, "I want to send you a little bit more information." I knew that he was highly educated, and I'd alluded to some studies when we were chatting. Later that night, I sent him three studies on low-back rehab and low-back performance.

Three days later, he called and asked to come in for a session. We spoke for about 20 minutes, and he bought a three-session package that I only agreed to after he got clearance from his doctor and was seen by a physical therapist. Those three sessions turned into a

20-session package, then three 50-session packages (at $4,500 each) for him and his girlfriend.

When I did the math, this one client amounted to over $20,000 in training from a single conversation and a follow-up email.

I asked him years later, when I was researching the updated version of *Ignite the Fire*, about why he hired me. He said, "You know, the conversation that we had was good. I was impressed by it, but what I was more impressed by is that you sent me follow-up information. You sent me stuff. You didn't pitch me. Nothing like that. You just sent me information, and said, 'Here, I hope that helps.'"[&]

So one conversation at a birthday party, where I wasn't pitching anybody, turned into $20,000 in revenue. If that doesn't convince you to improve your everyday communication skills, I don't know what will.

Marketing Method #2: Put Facebook to work for you

Facebook is nothing but a serendipitous machine that works for you, allowing you to keep in touch with a

---

Ignite the Fire was my first book. It is the most reviewed book for fit pros on Amazon and is widely regarded as "the Bible" for personal trainers. If you're liking this book, then you should also buy a copy of Ignite.

*& The paperback is available at **theptdc.com/ignite** and Kindle and audio versions are sold on Amazon.*

large number of people and broadcast messages to them. As you'll soon learn, there isn't one best way to use it to convert clients. Instead, use Facebook to foster as many loose connections as possible and, over time, increase your expert reputation with those connections.

If you set up your account properly, even within your small personal network, your chances of catching a lucky break go up simply by knowing somebody who knows somebody who has low-back pain and is looking for a trainer. That's what this is all about. That's how social media works in converting clients. It's not about direct ads to sales. It's about being top of mind with as many people as possible so that when they (or somebody they know) is interested in a trainer, you get the call.

That's why you can't determine the direct return on investment (ROI) of your Facebook activities. Paid advertising may be a small piece of the puzzle for you, but most of what you can use Facebook for is free and can't be measured or quantified because it happens in roundabout ways. For example, the number of potential clients who respond to paid ads is tiny when compared with how many will message their friends, "I'm thinking of hiring a trainer. Know anybody?" You need to put yourself in the position to get that message.

Hopefully you have been building up your Facebook network for years. If you don't have many connections, it's time to work on that.

I'll go over the process of systematically building your personal network on Facebook in a minute. First, a word on privacy and professionalism. If you are concerned about things like privacy, I suggest creating a secondary account that you use for close friends and family. (I have one, and it has about 45 connections).

For your new profile, individually message your close contacts and family members and ask them to join you there because you're going to make your existing profile more professional. Facebook policies state that you cannot use a personal profile for business. You're not. Instead, you're going to use it to create connections and relationships (exactly what Facebook is built for) and allow serendipity to run its course.

You can maintain a professional page in addition to your personal page if you like. This is where you'd keep it purely for business, get likes, send paid advertisements, etc. With your existing personal profile, the one that you've been building for years, you probably already have as many customers, clients, and contacts as you'll ever need.

You'll need to be the judge of whether it makes sense to go through your existing profile and delete any pictures and posts from your past that you deem unprofessional.* I left most of my pictures on my

---

*You know the ones I mean. As impressive as you were in your beer-chugging days in college, Frank the Tank, those photos will not impress potential clients.

Facebook page up, but I did make sure to trash the really bad ones.

Build Your Network: When you meet somebody, send a friend request. Go through your friend's friends lists and reconnect with people you knew back in the day. Search Facebook for high school and university connections. It's really that simple. People you once knew are people who have reason to trust you more than somebody they've never met. Over time, if you make it known that you're a fitness pro, you'll become the go-to expert and, when they or somebody they know are looking for a trainer, you've increased your chances of catching the lucky break and getting the call. This is how you manufacture serendipity.

Recall my two golden rules:

>*Do a great job.*

>*Make sure everybody knows about it.*

How will everybody know what a great job you do if you aren't connected to them? Connecting is the first step.

Over time, the power of this grows and it's impossible to measure. Your job then becomes simple: Post a health or fitness tip every day on Facebook. You can make a list of a bunch at once and post one a day or even hire an assistant or use software to automate the posting. It doesn't matter how it's done, just that it's done consistently.

You can also share materials from others with a quick thought about the material. You see, the goal is not necessarily to educate people. The goal is to stay top of mind with as many people as possible. To be the fitness person for them and their extended network.

Do this day in, day out. Grow your personal network on Facebook. Increasing your chances of that lucky break, and success, is always a matter of manufactured serendipity.[⚓]

Marketing Method #3: Harness mavens

The third piece of the puzzle is to build strategic relationships with the people who I call "secret neighborhood mavens." I learned about the concept of mavens in Malcolm Gladwell's classic book, The Tipping Point, and have taken it one step further to help you build a local personal training business.

A secret neighborhood maven is a well-connected person who holds influence in a network. Lots of books will tell you to connect with people like physicians, and, while this isn't a bad idea, physicians already have a lot of people trying to connect with them, their time is tight, and it's hard to figure out something you can offer a physician in exchange for referrals.

⚓ *I wrote an ebook called "Facebook Marketing for Fitness Pros" that goes into this in more detail. If you'd like a copy, go here:* **theptdc.com/facebook.**

The key to finding these secret mavens is to identify the folks in your neighborhood who interact with lots of potential clients over the course of a day, meet them on their own terms, and provide value to them. Here are the four best secret mavens that exist in almost every neighborhood:

Coffee Shop Baristas: Baristas serve people caffeine, so everybody loves them. The local coffee shop has local clientele who pick up a cup of joe (or mocha crappa frappa latte semi-hot with light foam for $8) every day as part of their routines. The maven barista knows the regulars by name, engages in daily small talk, and is loved. This person is also probably not paid a lot, works hard, and has one or more other interests outside of whipping up overpriced, obscurely complex caffeinated beverages.

To connect with the barista maven, you're going to be buying a lot of overpriced coffee. When you go to the local coffee shop, wear your trainer shirt. If you don't have a shirt with your company's logo that says "trainer" on it somewhere, then you can get a few printed from a website like CafePress. You'll pay about $20 a T-shirt, possibly less. You can even buy material to print yourself and iron onto an existing shirt.

On the first day, go in with a smile and ask the barista her name and leave a good tip. For the next week or two, go in at around the same time, greet the barista by name, and always wear your trainer's shirt. After a few days or weeks of this, calling the barista by her name, engaging in small talk, she'll ask you something like, "Hey, do you work at that gym down the street?"

At this point you tell her that you do, and offer a referral incentive if they send anybody your way. She'll probably say she's not allowed to do anything like that, but give her some of your cards anyway and ask if you can put a flyer up in the shop. Say something like, "Hey, if you meet anybody who says they may want training, be sure to send them my way." Then offer a referral of 10 percent of the first package a client buys from you. (Even if your gym doesn't support this, you can afford it).

Over time, baristas will start introducing you to other regulars — and you may get some calls, too, because they have your business cards. If you have some downtime, bring your computer or book and read there and just hang out. When I was training clients and writing for fitness magazines, I used to take my breaks and write in a local coffee shop, The Mad Bean in Toronto. Brian, the owner, often interrupted my writing and introduced me to other customers who he was chatting with because the conversations often revolved around health or fitness (as a lot of conversations tend to do).

The barista in a local coffee shop is a great connector in a small neighborhood. Baristas may not send you clients directly, but if you hang around long enough and become an easily accessible fitness and health information resource, they'll introduce you to others in the community and increase your odds of serendipity over time.

Hairdressers: Hairdressers' lives are full of small talk, and any business with a waiting area is a great place for you to leave some high-value materials. Hairdressers usually work independently (they rent chairs at salons) and don't make a lot of money. Offering them an opportunity to make a bit extra, for no additional work, always appeals.

Introduce yourself to the hairdressers during their downtime, usually between two to four p.m. Ask about their clientele, and offer to leave some reading material specific to their clientele, for the salon's waiting area. For example, one hairdresser I connected with had a lot of female clients in their 50s, 60s, and 70s, so I left material on postmenopausal fat loss. Write an article, or use an article written by someone else, and clip your business card to it.

Write a code on the business card that's specific to the hairdresser, and tell her that if anyone comes in as a result of the material or referrals, she'll get a referral incentive. When somebody mentions that code or that she was referred to you by that hairdresser, give the hairdresser a little kickback as thanks. (You might also consider referring people you know back to the hairdresser, too).

Every two to three weeks, pop into the salons in your area just to say hi to the hairdressers. Over time you want to build a tighter relationship with them. If you notice that their waiting area doesn't have a plant or flowers, consider bringing one as a gift. Anything that will set you apart.

Naturopathic Doctors/Holistic Practitioners: These professionals see a lot of people who are interested in preventive care and willing to spend money on it because their services are rarely covered in full by government or extended health care plans.

The process is generally the same as working with hairdressers. Ask about their clientele and if you can leave client-oriented material in their waiting area. You may also consider putting together a workshop for the neighborhood and co-presenting with the practitioner. It's a lot of work, but if you like presenting to small groups, it may be worth it.

Beyond that, follow the same process as you would with a hairdresser. Make yourself known, pop in from time to time to say hello, and give a gift to spruce up their office if you can.

Real Estate Agents: Real estate agents are the final secret mavens because they are the first point of contact for new people who move into the neighborhood. The biggest problem is that the good ones are super busy. You'll have to chase them. Some will respect your persistence because their business relies on that kind of thing.

To familiarize yourself with in-demand agents, go for a

walk. Using Google maps, create a perimeter for your neighborhood, pop on some good music, and walk around snapping pics of for-sale signs. You'll probably see two to three agents who are selling most of the houses in your area. Their office phone numbers will be on the sign. Call them, offer them two or three free sessions, or a free membership to the gym, if management allows.

It'll take a lot of follow-up. They'll probably say that they are too busy. If so, extend the offer to their spouse or child. Do your best to build a rapport with these real estate agents. An ideal situation: They include you as part of their "welcome" gift to new homeowners. Agents like to show that they know the best of the neighborhood. Make yourself their recommended source.

Marketing Method #4: Ask for referrals

The fourth way to market yourself with high integrity is to ask existing clients for referrals. It's common practice to offer something like a free session in exchange for a referral. I think that this is a terrible referral incentive. Clients are already training with you and willing to pay. Offer them something more personal. Say, "If you refer somebody, I'll give you a referral gift valued at up to $100."

When a client sends you a referral, give her something meaningful that shows you understand them. That may be the jersey of a favorite football player, or two tickets to the local opera because she mentioned she loves it. These gifts probably won't even cost $100 and will mean a lot more than a free session. It'll also help reinforce your relationship.

How to Ask a Client for a Referral: If you have spots open, take your client to your office and ask if she has two minutes to spare. Close the door behind her and say something like, "You know, Susie, I've had a few training spots open up, and I want to extend them to my clients' friends and family before marketing to the outside. I've really loved working with you. I was wondering if you know somebody who may benefit." If she says no, which may happen, thank her and say goodbye.

If she does know someone, probe for more info. What does this person want to achieve? Does she know of anything that may get in the way, like injuries? Some clients will open up with info about their friends or family members, and others won't. Either way, you want to give a takeaway, in the form of a card, letter, or coupon to pass along to this person she knows.

By the next day, your client has probably forgotten about your request. People are busy, right? Or he or she may have agreed to pass your name along to a friend but didn't really intend to. Asking clients again and again to get in touch with people can get awkward, and that's never good.

Instead, email your client the evening after you speak. Don't make it a hard sell. Just include some material (an article works well) related to the issue or goal that your client said her friend has. This gives your client an easy way to forward the email with your name attached. You can take it from there.

Asking her to pass along information is a nice way to bump her memory, and also give her an excuse to get in touch with her friend. Write something like, "Hey, thanks so much for talking to me about your friend. You know, I just came across this article, as I was thinking about her tonight, and I was hoping that you would pass it along for me." Odds are that your client will forward the message along with something like, "Hey, my trainer asked me to pass this along to you. I thought you may benefit from it." This is super-basic and just scratches the surface, but it can be effective. Hit send.

Marketing is manufacturing serendipity and adding value, not trickery

Remember, marketing doesn't mean manipulating people into doing things they don't want to do. Ethical marketing is simply identifying a need and figuring out ways to make yourself the go-to for that need, for as long as you need to, until somebody decides that they want to hire a trainer. When that happens, you'll have already positioned yourself as the obvious choice.

THE TAKEAWAY

You'll market yourself with integrity and attract clients when you focus on what you can do for them, and for the people who refer clients to you.

CHAPTER 10

Sell Your Training
Anatomy of a Perfect Sales Meeting

Selling is a skill. You don't need to be a salesperson or know all of the ins and outs of selling strategy (although that never hurts), but you do need to become proficient at sales.

If you have the right skills to help a client, your sales process starts and finishes with your ability to communicate how you can help him or her in a way that appeals to that person. It's that simple, and that hard.

Selling should never be scary. If you can help a client, you should want to sell him or her training. If you can't help, you should confidently tell that person that you aren't the best option.

Here's a story about how I didn't just lose a sale, but crashed and burned. I tell this story often because it illustrates so clearly how many trainers lose sales.

The Anatomy of a Bad Sales Meeting

Jeff was booked for a meeting with me by my manager. We hadn't yet met. When the day came, I said, "Hi," shook his hand, led him into an office, and asked him what his goal was.

>*—Pretty standard up until now.*

He told me he wanted to lose some weight, especially around his midsection. I nodded, pretended to listen, wrote it down (to show him that I was paying attention), and began to list my certifications.

>*— I did everything that I thought I should be doing but had already lost and didn't know it yet.*

As I proudly listed off my certifications and degree, I looked at his face for clues, hoping that he was appropriately impressed. He smiled and nodded.

>*— Ahh, the false smile and nod.*

After listing a whole bunch of certifications that meant nothing to him, I told Jeff that his problem was really his poor posture.

After my little talk, I asked Jeff for the sale. He said that he wasn't ready to buy a package yet because he needed to think about it.

>*— Nobody ever needs to think about it. If you hear*

this, it means that you either screwed up and said something that turned off the potential deal, or didn't address a quiescent objection. "I need to think about it" is the polite way of saying no.

I never heard from Jeff again.

What Went Wrong?

I want you to learn from my mistakes because I did three major things wrong:

1. **Fake listening**: I asked Jeff about his goals, and instead of listening, I spent the time thinking about how I was going to respond and impress him.
2. **Braggadociousness**: Jeff didn't care about my perceived overachievements. Neither my degree or my certifications meant anything to him because I didn't explain why they would help me help him.
3. **Proclamation**: Instead of listening to Jeff and educating him on weight loss, I was more interested in proclaiming that he also had a posture issue. I shouldn't have identified another problem. He was there for weight loss. Once I signed him on and gained his trust, I could have helped him deal with his posture issue, if it truly was an issue.

That was embarrassing. Let's talk about a good sales meeting now.

Here's a different sales meeting I had with a woman named Susie.

Similar to Jeff, I met her at the door with a smile and a
bottle of water. Making some small talk, I led her into
my office, offered her a seat, and asked about her goals.

Susie had some chronic shoulder pain. I asked her
more about it and, when ready to move on with the
conversation, I pulled out two articles from my file
in my desk, attached my business card to each, and
handed them to her while I continued to talk. "So you
have a bit of information about what may be going on,"
I said.*

Over the course of our conversation, Susie also told me
she lived far from the gym, and that travel may be an
issue. Before continuing, I wanted to nip this objection
in the bud, so I asked Susie whether I could tell her a
story of another client who had traveled to see me and
how I organized the schedule to make it work. She said
yes. I told the story. And she was ready to continue.

— The best way to deal with an objection is to relate a
story of how a client with a similar objection overcame
the problem.**

The rest of the meeting was pretty straightforward.
It took less than 30 minutes, much less time than my

---

* In an ideal world, you'll make the sale before a client leaves your office,
but that doesn't always happen. If possible, find an excuse to give a client
something to take along that reminds her of the conversation.

** In this case, the client and I met periodically for check-ins every
Saturday morning, and I kept my Saturday schedule open for this type of
training. (At the time, that's what I did. My Monday to Friday was sched-
uled every week, and then my Saturday morning was my program design
clients, and clients making up for lost time during the week if they'd been
sick or had to cancel).

meeting with Jeff, and Susie became a client. I didn't once mention my certifications, and I only mentioned my qualifications in relation to the two things that she cared the most about, which were shoulder rehab and working with clients who lived far from the gym.

The contrasting examples of my meetings with Jeff and Susie illustrate how important it is to focus on things clients care about. But don't think that sales skill is something that happens fast. It takes practice. These two examples were four years apart.

A sales meeting isn't a time to tell a client about everything you can do. Instead, a sales meeting is a time to ask the requisite questions to figure out what may stop the client from getting started so that you can get on with the most important part: the qualifications, experiences, and skills that will help the person overcome the issues that he or she is concerned about.

The four-step sales method

The following system for selling training is about as simple as you'll ever see. I've developed and field-tested (with tens of thousands of trainers in 82 countries) much more in-depth selling systems and scripts for my courses like the Online Trainer Academy certification program. However, to get you confident about selling, I want to keep this simple.

You want to sell to clients who are right for you, and that's what this system is designed to do. There are four steps. Each step represents one part of the sales meeting that will take you from your first encounter with the client to him handing over the credit card.

Step 1: *Assume control and dig deep.*

To start, ask a very basic, open-ended question like "What do you want to achieve?" Assuming and maintaining control of the conversation is going to be important all the way through. The best way is to always be the one asking questions.

After asking this, take notes as your future client talks. When he finishes and pauses, wait in silence for a count of two. Often, he'll speak again during this silent period because he or she wasn't finished.

If your client doesn't start to speak again after two seconds, and you're not satisfied with his answer, ask "Why?" You can ask "why" in a number of different ways depending on the situation, but the phrase, "Can you tell me a bit more about ...?" works really well.

Dig deeper, continuing to ask "why" until you're satisfied that you not only know what he wants to achieve, but why he wants to achieve it.

Once satisfied that you know the real "why," ask a few other requisite questions before continuing on to step 2:

- Medical history — Injuries, medical conditions, or aches and pains.

- Training history — Has the person worked with trainers before? If so, what did he like and not like?

- Training frequency — How often can he realistically work out each week (not necessarily with you.)

- Training interruptions — Are there any upcoming events in the next three months that may get in the way of training, like weddings, holidays, or other family events?

Before moving on to step 2, paraphrase back to the client what he just told you by saying, "Just to make sure that I'm 100 percent clear on what you're looking for, you want _____ and _____ but you're nervous about _____. Is that correct?"

This act of paraphrasing shows him that you were listening, that you understand what he wants and, more important, what he was nervous about. Write down the answers and move on to step 2.

Step 2: Sketch out a plan.

Give the client an idea of what the training would look like. Sketch out a plan that takes into account any limitations you've discussed — like planned breaks in training or injuries. This plan should give a general outline of the program and relate back to the reasons the client wants to exercise.

When you describe your program, use lines like, "Cool, Tony! To get you lean and mean for the summer, here's what I'm thinking..." At which point, you'll go over the basics of your plan.

A completely made-up example:

"Stage one will be the anatomical adaptation of the general preparation phase, where we prep your body for training. This will last two to three weeks, depending on how your body responds. Following that, I want to go through a full six-week hypertrophy, or muscle gain, phase. You see, muscle is metabolic, meaning that the more you have of it, the easier it will be to burn fat."

"So, even though your ultimate goal is to burn fat, packing on a little bit of muscle at the beginning will assist throughout the program as opposed to if we just did fat-burning the whole time. That leads me to the next stage, fat loss, where we'll be for four to six weeks. This is when your new muscle will really start to show up, as we shed some of the fat layer on top of it, making that T-shirt nice and snug just in time for summer. Or as I like to call it, T-shirt time. We'll call this the 'Sun's Out, Guns Out Workout.' "

Or whatever. I mean, obviously, this will change. What is important here is that you start to paint a picture of how things will go for the client to help him understand what he's going to be doing, and to help him envision himself doing it. You're also relating it back to his goals. The plan will never be perfect, and doesn't have to be, but it's a great place to get the client salivating about working with you and to explain some of the science to him.

Step 3: Address objections.

Objections are an opportunity to close. You want objections. The more objections, the better. If you somehow miss an objection, you'll lose the sale.

When you're done explaining the plan and relating it to his goals, simply ask, "How does that sound?" He may say "great" or "good." Or he may give you an objection or ask questions about the program.

It's okay to answer questions about the program and clarify anything that's unclear. If the client says the program sounds good, ask if he foresees anything that might get in the way of his progress before continuing. A sales meeting is really just a series of getting buy-ins and closing doors. After presenting the program, you want to ensure that this aspect of the deal is acceptable and understood before moving on.

By asking, "How does that sound?" you either get the verbal agreement that it's good (i.e., the buy-in), or a question to address. If at any point your client asks about cost, the best thing to say is that you offer a few different packages and aren't sure yet which is best. Have a printed piece of paper with your package options and hand it to the client saying, "Once we're done figuring out what you need, we can land on the best package."

Having the price sheet in his hands helps put the client at ease. You're not ready to discuss price, but you don't want to ignore the client's questions. You also don't want to give a price before you're ready to, because the cheapest trainer in the world is too expensive if you haven't sold the client on your value.

After you've handed over your sales sheet (if necessary), ask, "Okay, are you ready to continue?" Once he says yes, continue by asking if he has any other questions. When the client says no, ask, "Is there anything else you think could get in the way of training?"

This process of closing all objection windows before you ask for the sale is necessary so that hidden objections you failed to deal with don't bite you in the butt later. If your client brings up another objection, deal with it and repeat, "Is there anything else that you think could get in the way of your training?" Repeat this until the client says no.

Now that the objection window is closed, get the client to buy into the schedule before bringing up price. You have your ballpark training plan already, so mock up a schedule and hammer out the days and times that the client will train. A line as simple as, "Great! So, at twice a week, I have Wednesdays and Fridays available mid-afternoon, at two to three p.m. Do those times work for you?" Figure out a few slots that work for him and get him to say yes. Then ask for the sale.

Step 4: Get the buy-in (and talk money).

This should be as simple as asking for a credit card and taking payment, but it's not always straightforward.

Now that you've gotten everything else out of the way, it's time to discuss money and relate it back to his goals. You may say something like, "Well, Tony, based on what we've talked about, I think that seeing me twice a week and working out on your own twice a week is what you need to achieve your goal of _____. I'll guide you on what to do when you're training without me and review your progress."

As you talked with the client, you should've already chosen two packages — your first and second choices. Always present one option as better than the other, but say that there is a second option available. You may say, "Now, the most cost-effective package is option one. But if that's too much to commit to right now, then option two is a great choice, as well. Also, remember that no matter what, there's a full guarantee on any unused sessions. Are you ready to get going?"

Giving the client two options takes it from a yes or no decision to an A or B decision. Instead of the client asking, "To train or not to train?" he's now asking, "Should I take option A or option B?" Always suggest the best option for the client to help him decide, and I recommend offering the guarantee on any unused sessions. Unfortunately, it's common for someone to have had a bad experience with the fitness industry, like being ripped off by another trainer.

Offering a guarantee helps offset these kinds of experiences. Say something like, "No matter what — if you move away or whatever — there's a full guarantee on the sessions. We'll refund your money, no questions asked."

After you say, "Are you ready to get going?" be quiet. You've made the ask. New or unconfident trainers will get nervous when they make the ask and try to fill the silence by talking about the program more.

At this point, you've said everything you need to say. It's time for your client to respond. It may take a couple of seconds. Bite your lip. Do whatever you have to do. It's the client's turn to speak.

A few things may happen, and I want to talk about each of them in turn. If your client says yes, cool. You're done. Draw up the paperwork, and schedule the client in. Good job.

Still, this is the point when other objections may come up. Sometimes the objection is a window you failed to close during the sales meeting. Other times the objection isn't the real objection — it's masking another issue that the client, for some reason, isn't willing to come out and say.

A primer on objections

What if the client objects to something other than price? Maybe he'll say that he's not sure if he has the time to commit or he needs to get a shoulder injury checked out first. If this happens, you missed dealing with that objection earlier in the sales process. You failed to close the objection window. It's not a huge deal most of the time, but get past the objection immediately and make sure you don't make that mistake again.

What follows is a primer on how to deal with the most common objections. This primer also appears in the *Personal Trainer Pocketbook: A Handy Reference for All Your Daily Questions.* Included in this section are:

1. The "what does it cost?" objection.
2. The "previous injury" objection.
3. The "bad experience with a previous trainer" objection.
4. The "I have to ask my spouse/partner" objection.
5. The "too expensive" objection.
6. The "no time" objection.
7. The "I have to think about it" objection.

1. The "what does it cost?" objection

In any sales meeting, you want to avoid making a proposition until you've had a chance to build a rapport with the person, communicate the specific value to him, and deal with any objections. But I get it. Clients will

---

* The Personal Trainer Pocket Book is a handy guide with 48 answers to the 48 most common problems and situations that arise over the course of a trainer's day. While it can be read start-to-finish, it's better used as a reference, kept on hand so that whenever a question arises, you can flip to the corresponding page, find the answer, and navigate the problem well.

You can get the book in paperback directly from our store at **theptdc.com/store** *or on Kindle from Amazon.*

ask how much training costs before you've had a chance
to do all those things.

First, I suggest publishing all prices on your website.
This way people can check in advance. I know that
when I go shopping, I avoid stores that don't list
prices. There's a comfort level in knowing how much
something costs before going in. In not publishing
prices on your website, you're silently suggesting you're
very expensive or, worse, that you're hiding your prices
for some deliberate sales reason. Either way, you're
turning people off and missing out on countless leads.

Still, in a meeting, try to avoid the cost question. You
want clients understanding full value before they
hear final cost. First, try to deflect it. If at any point
someone asks how much your training costs, say, "I'd
like to understand more about your goals before we talk
money, if that's okay," and ask another question.

If he still presses you for price, there's not much
you can do other than present the options. Have a
professional rate sheet printed and put it on the table
so you can both see it. Tell him there are options, but
that you truly don't know what's best until you ask a
few more things — but he's welcome to hold on to it for
the time being. Then continue your conversation.

Rule #1 is to make the client feel comfortable. Rule
#2 is to give yourself an opportunity to get all of the
information that you need and say what you need to
say before making a sales proposition. In giving your

client the rate sheet to "hold on to," you make her feel more comfortable and can continue the conversation as planned.

2. The "previous injury" objection

Above all, make sure you understand the injury. I suggest keeping a database on the most common injuries you come across. (When you come across a new injury, make sure to add it to the database). Also keep articles and papers describing the injury and rehabilitation protocols.

If you're familiar with the injury, proceed to pummel the client with knowledge, so to speak. If you're not familiar with the injury, use the line, "I can help you with that." Proceed to take notes on the injury, and do further research after the client has left to determine whether you can deal with it or who to refer out to.

Either way, your goal is to have information in your file to offer the client as a takeaway (with your business card stapled to it, of course).

3. The "bad experience with a previous trainer" objection

Never, ever bad-mouth anybody. Always give a former trainer the benefit of the doubt, but educate the client as to how you would treat the situation differently. Say the client didn't feel the previous trainer listened to her.

I would tell her I was sorry about that, and as my client, she can call me during the day or email me anytime.

Whatever the bad experience was, show that you're going to be different, and better. Be specific and don't move on until you have shown her that you won't repeat the same mistake her previous trainer made.

4. The "I have to ask my spouse/partner" objection

Tough one. So tough that I've yet to come across a single effective method to deal with this objection. Because of that, I suggest proactively dealing with it. When setting up the sales meeting, ask the client if she has "anybody else who may be involved in the decision-making process." This way he or she will hopefully bring his or her partner to the sales meeting and, as a result, the objection won't come up.

5. The "too expensive" objection

If you've demonstrated your value to a potential client, cost shouldn't be an obstacle.

Yes, some people can't afford a trainer, but the fact that you're a little cheaper or more expensive than another trainer shouldn't matter. If $80/hour is too expensive, so is $70. But if a client understands your value, she won't balk at $80/hour.

If cost comes up as an objection, first revisit all the other objections and ensure they're all properly dealt with (cost often acts as the fallback if something else is an issue). If the client still objects to the price, stay quiet for five seconds or so. Often she will talk herself into the sale. If that's not happening, present a more cost-effective option, offer an extended payment plan, or wish her well and stay in touch.

6. The "no time" objection

If a client says she doesn't have time to train, discuss different workout routines suited to her goals that will work within her timeline. For example, if you have a client who wants to lose fat, discuss metabolic workouts and how much more "bang for your buck" these workouts will get her as opposed to steady-state cardio.

There are many ways to alter a workout to hit a specific goal. If there's any way for you to break up the programming so it fits her schedule while still keeping the goal in mind, do it. This could include telling your client that home workouts will be required, for example. If there's really no way for you to change the programming to meet her time constraints, be honest. If you're up-front and say that her goals require more time and you're not willing to train her under any other circumstances, I've found that clients usually make the time.

7. The "I have to think about it" objection

This isn't an objection. What does the client need to think about? Ask her and be quiet. There's always a tangible reason behind this objection. Don't be satisfied until she gives you a tangible answer.

CHOOSE CAREFULLY: YOU DON'T WANT TO SELL EVERY CLIENT

I can't give you a system that guarantees a sale every time because, frankly, you don't want to sell every client. You've got space to train maybe 15 to 20 a week, at one to three weekly sessions. That's not a lot of customers. You should choose your clients just as much as they choose you.

A sales meeting is a time to learn about what the client wants to achieve, how committed he is, and how realistic his goals are with any financial or time limitations that he may have. If there's going to be an issue, better to figure it out before you begin than find out later. This way you can either create a plan that works within the constraints of the client's limitation or tell him honestly that you aren't the right solution for him.

Refusing to take money from somebody you cannot help is not only the right way to do business; it could also drive business as well.

In my days training clients, I often turned away business. For example, if a client honestly couldn't afford to work with me consistently, I'd tell him not to buy three sessions because he would get just as much from a workout in a book. I would be happy to do a session with a client to show him how to safely perform the exercises in the program but would be happier for him to save his hard-earned money. Whenever this happened, the result was one of three things:

The client now believed me when I said that what I could offer was special and became willing to do more sessions with me.

The client did what I said and bought a workout and became a friend in the gym who trusted me explicitly, telling other members how great I was and recommending me to friends and family, resulting in referrals.

The client did what I said and bought a workout. Or didn't — but I slept better at night knowing that I did the right thing.

I bring this same mentality to my current business of educating trainers. Each time we open enrollment to the Online Trainer Academy Certification Program, we turn away dozens of potential students ready to buy.

I'll never forget an email I got from the husband of a woman who spoke to my team on live chat. This man was so impressed that we actually cared about his wife enough to tell her not to spend her money because the course wasn't right for her that he was going to encourage her to become a lifelong customer of ours. I checked, and she enrolled in our next period when she was truly ready for the course.

If you sell to every client, you may make a few extra sales, but you'll end up training a whole bunch of people you shouldn't be working with. Not only does this drain your energy, but you're in this for the long-term. Personal training gets to be a darn fun job when you've built a reputation based on trust.

This is personal training sales. There's nothing "scammy" here. You're not tricking anybody to do anything they don't want to do. Selling happens when you put yourself in the best position possible to help the client, if you can. And if you can't, well, you can't, and there's nothing wrong with that either.

THE TAKEAWAY

A simple sales process will help you connect with clients, convince them to hire you, and build a rock-solid business and reputation based on trust.

CHAPTER 11

Goose Your Bottom Line

How to Make More Money as a Trainer

At the start of your career, you may be concerned about your primary income from training clients and how you can increase it. As your career progresses, you'll need to figure out a way to make money while not training clients on the floor. Training is a service business and, as with any service business, you'll eventually develop a bottleneck and your income will hit a ceiling.

Follow the guidelines in this book and you'll increase your earning potential, enabling you to raise your rates, but the time will come when you simply cannot charge any more, or work any harder.

This chapter is about leveraging your expertise, reputation, and intellectual property to boost your income. How to do all that? By developing multiple, varied, and passive income streams. Fun stuff, and it's easier than you think. But what I'm about to say comes with a warning: Your integrity and reputation always come first. No amount of money is worth sacrificing either.

The first part of this chapter will discuss ways to boost your worth and position yourself to make more cash in the future. The second part deals with specific opportunities available to you.

Education and network come first

When I first started training clients full-time, I was reasonably successful. After a short while, I had a full stable of clientele, but my income painted a bleak picture. At 30 to 40 client hours per week, I was making just over $35,000 a year after taxes. Thirty to forty client hours generally equates to 50 to 65 hours in the gym. That made for long days.

Each day started early and ended late. A social life was out of the question. For a 21-year-old, this was fine. But after a few years, I figured that at some point I may want a family. If that was going to happen, something had to change. And if that was going to happen, it was up to me.* Not knowing much about business at that time, I figured that if I became better at it, I'd increase

---

* And if I wanted a family, it probably meant that I needed a girlfriend. And if I wanted a girlfriend, it probably meant that I needed the time and energy to go on a date or two or three.

my value and the money would flow. So I read.

With no background and no idea where to look, I grabbed my brother's first-year university marketing textbook off the shelf (I was living in my parents' basement at the time) and read it cover to cover. Next I headed to the local bookstore with a pen and paper and wrote down the names of bestselling books and authors in the marketing category. The library was next door to the bookstore, so, list in hand, I began checking out the books on, or related to, my list.

There's no shortcut or hack to this stuff. It takes time. Back then I didn't have money to hire a coach or mentor or sign up for an expensive course. Fortunately, most knowledge is free. Courses and coaches are valuable because they save you time. But when you don't have money, you need to trade time. Once you have a bit of money, you'll begin systematically buying back your time at a discount. But I'm getting ahead of myself.

Earlier in this book, I shared my rule for reading that was developed way back when I was checking books out of the library. Every night, Monday to Friday, I read for a minimum of an hour. If I missed time, I made up for it on the weekend.

It's hard for me to explain what happened next because it was quick and a blur, and hindsight is 20/20. What I do know is that it didn't take long for me to leapfrog all of my peers in clientele, income, and earning potential.

I was a good-enough trainer and my clients liked me, and now, armed with the skillset of a marketer, opportunities seemed endless. As you develop a better business acumen, you'll begin seeing opportunities everywhere that others seem to miss.

An example: The book *Linchpin* by Seth Godin had a big impact on me. I've gifted this book more than any other. Before reading it, I saw myself as just another trainer. The book taught me the importance of going above and beyond in times when I wasn't asked, making myself indispensable to the organization that I was working for. When you do that, Godin argued, you're in control and can command higher income and a better working environment.

There wasn't anything major, but, after reading that book, I started looking for opportunities to help out. Sometimes it was small stuff like picking up garbage around the gym. Other times I'd offer to put on a continuing education seminar for my colleagues by presenting on a book that I was reading. I took it on myself to call Lululemon and do demonstrations in their office on behalf of the gym, networked with local businesses, and so much more. The result was an influx of demand for my services and a unique position in my club.

By the time I was 23, my take-home pay had almost doubled from $25 an hour to $41.80 an hour. Not only that, I got promoted to senior trainer and began earning a base salary, and was put in charge of mentoring other trainers. I also snagged commissions from referring my overload of clients to other trainers.

By becoming more valuable as a result of this studying, I was able to work fewer hours and make just as much, or more, than before. In the years that followed, I decreased my hours from 40 to 25 hours per week and continued to train 20 to 25 clients a week for a few more years.

Having more time enabled me to write my first book, *Ignite the Fire* (available at **theptdc.com/store**), and start a website. Now, a few short years later, I have a healthy combination of income streams, many of them passive, and a business that allows me to control my own schedule to spend ample time with my wife and newborn son. And it all started with dedication to study and self-improvement, an hour a day, Monday to Friday.

It's not sexy. Most won't do it. That's why you should. [⚭]

Determining your time value

In the previous section, I hinted that as you begin to make more money, you can start to buy your time back at a discount. Knowing how much your time is worth makes it easy to figure out when it's a good idea to pay money to save time.

What follows is a process that I speak about in a few of my books and in *The Fundamentals of Online Training*

⚭ *I maintain an up-to-date list of the best business and marketing books for personal trainers here: **theptdc.com/book-list**.*

textbook that comes along with the Online Trainer Academy certification program. It's that important.

You can easily estimate the value of your time, per hour. As your career progresses, revisit this exercise because the numbers and ramifications will change.

The most obvious way would be to calculate your hourly rate and use that. But your hourly rate is not an accurate estimate of your time because it doesn't include a lot of the other things you must do, like:

- Travel to and from the gym
- Client research
- Program writing
- Administrative work
- Client file maintenance
- Anything else that could be confidently categorized as "work"

Your time value is the total amount of money that you make after taxes per year divided by the actual amount of hours it takes you to earn that money. You may be surprised at how little per hour you make. [&]

Armed with your time value, you can begin the process of buying back your time. If you can spend less money than the value of that time based upon your calculations, then it's a smart investment to buy it

*& For a more in-depth process of figuring how much your time is worth at any one time, down to the cent, read this: **theptdc.com/time-value**.*

back. This may mean taking a taxi over the bus, hiring an assistant to help out with administrative work, or paying somebody to clean or cook for you (or a host of other things). As long as you're filling the hours that you're now saving with productive tasks, you've made a good investment.

The point is that over time, the best investment you can make is in yourself. Knowing your time value allows you to confidently know the best time to make those investments.

No matter how you do it, making more money will require you to invest time into building a reputation that precedes you, business development, and/or crafting intellectual property to sell. These are three direct ways to make more money, so let's talk about each.

Reputation and your true value

Previously in this book, I told you that being able to find your own clients can help you increase your hourly rate, which means more money. But to what end? Making more per hour is great for a while, but you're still trading time directly for money and will eventually need to get off that hamster wheel. Your true value has little to do with writing programs and training clients.

The industry is one of the most profitable in the world, and you are at its forefront. So you need to develop two important assets: Creating a reputation, and assembling a group of people who trust your recommendation enough to buy stuff when you ask them to. Advertisers and promoters of everything from fitness equipment to food to supplements to books and cookbooks to videos will be banging down your door, wanting to pay you money for access to your audience.

To take advantage of this, I urge you to shift your mindset and recognize the value of your word, your knowledge, your network, and, ultimately, your reputation. While you may think more of things like Facebook and LinkedIn when I speak of networks, personal networks, like your friends and family, can be just as valuable. You can build your network with something as simple as sending a random email to a friend you haven't spoken to in years to check in.

While blogging or creating videos to grow your platform and brand are fantastic, these things are daunting and can take time, which you may or may not have. To start, I advise keeping it simple. You're reading and learning and growing already, so why not create a simple website and Facebook page with the goal of sharing what you're learning. This could be your study notes, made public for the world. Don't worry about promoting or even if anybody is paying attention. Instead, just keep putting it out day after day. Like getting in shape, the way to grow a platform is simple; it's just not easy.

In addition to sharing what you're learning, be eager to share materials from others in the industry who you support or are learning from. The more the better.

Curation — taking the time to bring together the best resources — is valuable for readers. Curate the best stuff you come across and you quickly become the center of an information network.

Be careful when using your reputation to make more money

With great reputation comes great responsibility. Owning a platform and having people who trust your recommendation leads to a host of revenue-generating opportunities. The caveat before going further is that no amount of money is worth risking the reputation that you painstakingly built. It takes a lifetime to build a rep and seconds to destroy it.

As time goes on there will be a host of "opportunities" presented to you. Often, the person trying to recruit you will even refer to it as an opportunity. Think very long and hard and do your research before deciding to sell things like food and supplements. There is nothing inherently wrong with multilevel marketing programs, supplement reseller programs, and canned fitness programs. But many of the products are overpriced and low-quality, and the programs prey on new trainers, selling them on a dream, leaving the majority of them with less money than they started with and tarnished personal relationships resulting from the pressure to sell to family and friends.

I'm not saying you shouldn't sell these things. All I'm saying is that I urge you to do your own research before you make a decision on whether, and what, to sell. In the beginning of this book, you learned about the importance of being able to do your own research and draw your own conclusions about any claims that people make. That means you do more than read the studies and materials the companies give you. Do some detective work.

Also, consider if the thing you're selling is offered at an appropriate price. Often, supplements or other products are priced much higher than they should be to make up for the large commissions. As a result, your customers suffer. And what happens when your customers find out that they had to pay a lot more for the product because you got a large commission?

There's a reason why almost every significant multilevel marketing company in the fitness and health industry has lost at least one large class-action lawsuit for millions of dollars. I'm not saying that they're all bad, but I urge you to be very careful.

Every trainer needs a blog

Starting a blog changed my life, so I'm biased. As I mentioned earlier, it's a great place to journal as you learn. It's also an opportunity to improve your writing. There's no need to put any undue pressure on yourself to learn how to become a blogger. What matters is that you put your thoughts out into the world, at least to start.

A blog, which can be standalone or part of a bigger website, is where potential clients will check you out before meeting you. Not having one could mean losing clients that you never even knew existed. Simply having a place where people can find out more about you before having to get on the phone or email you means that they'll feel more at ease when they finally talk to you.

Fitness blogs create fitness experts. An expert wields the power of his or her audience. Once you become an expert, your reputation becomes valuable and, as a result, it becomes easier to develop multiple income streams, many of which I'll discuss in the coming pages.

There are two types of fitness writers: innovators and simplifiers. An innovator lives on the cutting edge of research. This likely isn't you. A simplifier takes complex fitness information and makes it accessible to either the masses or a specific segment of the population. Simplifiers make up the majority of popular blogs. You're writing for your desired clients, not to impress other trainers. You don't need to write things to blow people away.

A blog by itself is almost never an income stream. You can probably make a few pennies with advertising, but website advertising revenue has dwindled for all but a few massive websites with many millions of page views. Instead, your blog will serve as a place to attract and gather an audience, small or big. From it, you can make money through the ways described on the following pages. Having a blog isn't necessary for anything I'm about to say, but it helps.

Let's move on to the different revenue streams available to you as a respected fitness professional.

Consider Affiliate Programs

Commission, partner, or affiliate programs are a fantastic way to start making a few extra dollars by recommending products or services that you believe can benefit your clients. Almost every major company has some sort of an affiliate program. They all work the same way:

> —*You sign up as an affiliate or partner and get a custom link.*

> —*If somebody clicks on the company's website through your link and buys something, you get paid.*

What's more, many of these links include something called cookies. This way, the person doesn't even have to buy when he first clicks on the link. As long as he clicks through to the website through your link and buys something within a predetermined period, you get paid.

If you have a blog, you can easily embed links in your articles. These links sit there forever and if anybody ever clicks on them and buys, you make money. If you don't have a blog or website, you can still email a link to a client when you make a recommendation.*

Amazon is the most common affiliate company. After registering as an Amazon Associate (its name for affiliate), you can get a custom link to any product on the site. So if you write a blog post and you link out to a book or supplement or piece of fitness equipment, and somebody goes to Amazon and buys the product, you get a percentage of the sale (and anything else that they buy) in your account.

A lot of fitness equipment or supplement companies work the same way. After registering for their affiliate program, you get a custom link, embed it on your site, share on social media, or email it along, and, if somebody buys, you get a percentage of the sale.

Generally the highest potential for revenue comes in the form of e-books and online information products. Commissions on sales are often in the 50 to 75 percent range. So you could write a blog post about cooking, for example, and link to a cookbook you like that includes video lessons and sells for $67. If somebody buys through your link, or somebody clicks through your link and then buys, four months later you'll get about $48 for every single sale. This is about 75 percent, minus payment processing fees for a single sale. If 10 people buy, that's almost $500 for a single link.

Get the idea? Now imagine if you have an archive of material, all with links to different products sitting

* *The Federal Trade Commission (FTC) requires you to disclose that you are getting paid a commission if the person buys.*

there. If people buy, you get paid. It doesn't take many sales to generate a nice supplement to your income, does it?

Every time someone comes to your site, you have the opportunity to make money from affiliate links. If your site gets any traffic from search engines, you may get an affiliate sale. If you link to an old article through your Facebook, you may get an affiliate sale. If somebody asks you a question, and you link to an article, you may get an affiliate sale. Even if somebody is looking for a cookbook, and you recommend it directly, sending them your unique link, you can get that commission. And it's easily an extra $50 or $100, or even many hundreds or thousands of dollars per week. You just need to do your due diligence and compile a list of products, services, and books that you would stake your reputation on.

Online training: Already the next big thing

Since online training became a part of the mainstream fitness industry, I've arguably been the most vocal advocate of it. So much so that I literally wrote the textbook on the subject, The Fundamentals of Online Training, and my team and I created the world's first certification program for online trainers called the Online Trainer Academy.

> *The Online Trainer Academy is the first-ever certification for online training. I've mentioned it a few times in this book. Upon enrolling, you receive a package in the mail that includes the seminal textbook,* The Fundamentals of Online Training; *your workbook; and access to the digital portal with video lessons, scripts, done-for-you templates, and more.*
>
> *To learn more about how you can boost your credentials and reclaim your life by becoming a certified online trainer, go to* **theptdc.com/ota**.

Online training is a sensational way for great trainers to make more in less time with a better schedule. I don't view it as a way to magically make boatloads of cash with very little work. It's a tool to take back control of your own schedule, your career, and your life. It creates space.

In some instances, coaches will scale it and make hundreds of thousands of dollars, but in most cases this extra time will be invested into family, writing a book, volunteering more, pursuing a hobby, or whatever your definition of freedom is.

Training clients in a gym can leave you exhausted because you aren't in control. No matter how great a job you do, you'll still be at the mercy of everything from the gym owner's mood to your clients' schedules, to weather and traffic, and a host of other things.

When it comes to creating an accessory income stream, it's a nice thought to write an e-book and sell thousands of copies passively. It's a good dream to have to develop a transformation program where you take 50, 100, or more paying clients through the program at once, scaling yourself substantially. The reality is that, for most, these things are only possible with a tremendous up-front outlay of time and money.

That time and money has to come from somewhere, and the best somewhere I know is slowly incorporating an online training component in your business. It could be purely online, or hybrid online-offline. Five to 10 online clients could mean an extra $500 to $3,000 a month, more than enough for you to better organize your in-person training schedule and commit that extra time and mental energy into whatever big audacious project you're dreaming of (or just be happy with the extra revenue and take more time with the people you love).

The point is, with online training as part of your services, you take back control. My definition of wealth is synonymous with freedom. It's up to you to dictate your own life, whatever that means to you. Online training is the first step, after you've gained some experience with your in-person clientele, toward that freedom.

Leading workshops

If you like to present, you can also lead workshops, both online and in person. The best part is that you do the work once to build this workshop or presentation, and then charge a premium for presenting the materials time and time again. You can offer the workshop live in your neighborhood to make extra money and attract new clients. Or you can offer it online — software like GoToWebinar will allow you to charge a fee for people to attend your workshop, and/or get access to the recording.

You can present on anything from fat loss to muscle gain to something more nuanced like fat-loss considerations for postmenopausal women. The benefit of this is that if you do have a website or blog, you can create an hour-long or two-hour presentation that you then charge $20 or $30 to access. Create it once and never touch it again.

Writing for publication

If you blog, you may also want to consider writing for pay. This can be a nice add-on because of the exposure. Having a few extra bucks never hurts, but you won't make a lot writing for pay unless you become well-known or prolific. Writing for other people should be seen less as an income stream and more as a way to drive traffic to your site, create a bigger audience for your business, or make some nice bonus cash.

THE TAKEAWAY

There are many ways to make money as a trainer. Just make sure that when you decide to pursue one, you do the homework to protect your reputation.

The End, but Really the Beginning

This book didn't tell you what to do. If that's what you were looking for, then I apologize. At this stage in your career, it would have been a disservice for me to pretend that I knew all the right answers for you. Because of that, the goal of this book was to teach you how, not what, to think.

A career in fitness comes with lots of questions, no set answers, and endless possibilities. Your days will sometimes be long, and when they're done, your feet will be sore and armpits sweaty. From time to time you may feel frustrated that you don't know enough or that others seem to have all the success. Never forget that you're now in an industry where you get to change lives for a living. It's fun.

So this is the end of the book. But, for you, it's the beginning of your fitness career, and I'm glad that you're here with us.

—*Coach Jon*

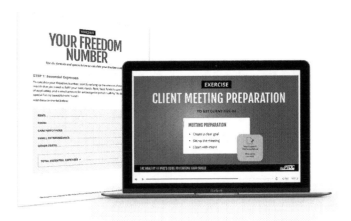

YOU'VE READ THE BOOK.
NOW ACE THE TEST.

And get the CECs/CEUs to prove it!

We want the Wealthy Fit Pro Guides to be your definitive resources for career and business success. That's why we've designed exclusive short courses based on each WFPG. Not only will you gain a deeper understanding and application of the material in this book, you'll also earn continuing education credits from your certifying organization — guaranteed.

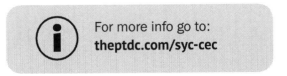

For more info go to:
theptdc.com/syc-cec

These courses are guaranteed to meet all of the requirements for you to gain CECs / CEUs from every certifying body. Even if your certification is not on the pre-approval list, you'll receive a pdf with detailed instructions on how to receive credit from your cert. If you aren't approved for any reason, we'll give you a full refund for the course.